Understanding BRCA

Living with the breast cancer gene

Highly Commended, 2018 BMA Book Awards
Winner, Beryl Bainbridge First Time Author Award, 2019

In memory of my mum

***

James, Isabelle and Ben; I love you so much.
You are everything I've ever wanted and you have given me
so much happiness

Understanding BRCA

Living with the breast cancer gene

Clarissa Foster

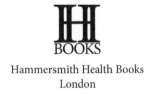

Hammersmith Health Books
London

First published in 2017 by Hammersmith Health Books – an imprint of
Hammersmith Books Limited
4/4A Bloomsbury Square, London WC1A 2RP, UK
www.hammersmithbooks.co.uk

Reprinted 2018, 2021, 2023

The information contained in this book is for educational purposes only.
It is the result of the study and the experience of the author. Whilst the
information and advice offered are believed to be true and accurate at
the time of going to press, neither the author nor the publisher can ac-
cept any legal responsibility or liability for any errors or omissions that
may have been made or for any adverse effects which may occur as a
result of following the recommendations given herein. Always consult a
qualified medical practitioner if you have any concerns regarding your
health.

British Library Cataloguing in Publication Data: A CIP record of this
book is available from the British Library.

Print ISBN 978-1-78161-120-3
Ebook ISBN 978-1-78161-121-0

Commissioning editor: Georgina Bentliff
Designed and typeset by: Julie Bennett, Bespoke Publishing Ltd.
Cover design by: Julie Bennett, Bespoke Publishing Ltd.
With photograph by: Ravinder Crone
Author photo by: Andy Ginger
Index: Dr Laurence Errington
Production: Helen Whitehorn, Path Projects Ltd.
Printed and bound by: TJ Books Limited.

Contents

Forewords

In this book, Clarissa presents the most thorough overview of a BRCA patient's journey. Her story starts years before she realised she might be a BRCA carrier with her own mother's diagnosis of ovarian cancer and covers the decades from her teens to her 30s. She combines the most personal of stories with detailed facts about all manner of issues, including meeting a genetic counsellor, the surgical options available to BRCA carriers which reduce risk and how the various surgeries have affected her physical, social and psychosexual wellbeing. Whether you have just been diagnosed as being a BRCA carrier, know someone affected or suspect you might be considered high risk, this book offers a wealth of information, interspersed with one lady's incredibly brave journey.

Niki Petrie, Consultant Plastic & Reconstructive Surgeon

I remember first meeting Clarissa in a busy clinic one Friday morning. In the short time allocated for her appointment, we discussed a whole myriad of life-changing and irreversible decisions that she faced because of the BRCA gene mutation that she possessed. We discussed the pros and cons of risk-reducing breast surgery, and although the options were all supported by a wealth of useful associations and statistics, none told the whole story and none told Clarissa exactly what to do. It was apparent from that first meeting that Clarissa had a scientifically trained mind and was balancing the evidence for and against each of her choices. Consultations for risk-reducing surgery are slightly different from other consultations, because the disease has not appeared yet and, indeed, may never do so. Logic and rational thought are needed, but because the science is incomplete, the logic becomes increasingly hazy the deeper you dig. It resembles a half-finished jigsaw puzzle, from which we can only deduce the final picture: and that deduction is personal, because we all see the puzzle in a slightly different light. It is that emotional interaction with the facts that makes us unique. For example: what does a 30% chance of getting a disease actually mean to any one person? To them personally, they either are going to get the disease (100%) or not (0%). Furthermore, how do you correlate the risk reduction with the risks of surgery and a permanently altered body? If there is a 30% chance of something happening and we operate on 100 people, then 30 of those people will have benefited, but 70 will have had the procedure unnecessarily. How does that affect a patient's thoughts and emotions? Clarissa has made that journey.

In many respects this book mirrors our consultation. Clarissa has assembled the facts and figures and taken the interpretations and assumptions as far as the incomplete science allows. Incomplete because the science is constantly being advanced and treatments are always changing. Incomplete because we are making lifelong decisions based on fragmented data. Incomplete because the follow-up of previous patients never includes everyone; people move, people forget, other things happen to them. Incomplete, because in the next few years all these decisions could be rendered unnecessary by the advent of a new preventative therapy. But this book tells us how it is today and patients reach a point when they have to make real decisions today, not next year. Time is often a luxury they cannot afford, so they have to put thoughts of the future to one side. Choices have to be made and then acted upon, with all their consequences.

This is what makes this book a 'must read' for anyone facing these choices. They have the knowledge that something may happen to them, often something that patients have witnessed in their loved ones, but crucially may also not happen to them. The risk-reducing treatments that we offer today are significant. The tools of my trade (as a plastic and reconstructive surgeon) are very unforgiving and the risk of complications adds another layer of complexity to already difficult decisions. I am always struck by how brave my patients are prior to surgery and also the importance of support from family and friends. This book is so informative to those who support patients too because Clarissa has given us a summary of the literature as it is today and then shared the emotional journey that she and her loved ones went through.

Although each patient's journey is unique, we are all human and anyone carrying a BRCA gene mutation will probably go on a remarkably similar journey. A shared approach to risk reduction involving patients and their doctors is essential. Reading this book places the patient and their family support in an ideal position to achieve that. Bravo, Clarissa.

Mike Tyler, Consultant Plastic & Reconstructive Surgeon

The BRCA mutations are the second most common cancer-causing genes that we can inherit. Identifying people who have these mutations and helping them manage their risk is a hugely important part of keeping people healthy and preventing avoidable cancers.

Clarissa has written a highly accessible and informative book that reflects not just her scientific background but also her experience as someone who has watched a loved one die of a cancer caused by a mutation and as someone who knows they are carrying a gene that can do this to them. She has written this book with the same approach that she used to make her own decisions. She has sought out all the information that's available, not just by reading and researching but also by talking with doctors experienced in looking after people carrying mutations and preventing and treating the cancers they get. Her advisors have included not just those of us who counselled and treated her but others who have generously given time to make sure their areas of expertise are also fully represented.

In this way, Clarissa has achieved the most accurate and comprehensive review of what we know about BRCA mutations currently available anywhere. But whilst it is detailed in its medical content it requires no real background knowledge to understand. It is written for everyone. Clarissa has ordered and analysed the evidence and asked probing questions. She has taken nothing for granted and I know from my many discussions with her that every guideline and research conclusion has been asked to justify itself. In medicine we know that we still have to make decisions even when there is doubt. So it is for women and men carrying these mutations. But she has done more than that. She has opened up and shared her own experiences in intimate detail. And this gives a real human context to the science so that anyone reading this book for help will know that they are not alone. Others have shared the distress and faced the same anxieties but taken control of their destiny and come out the other side stronger and more positive.

I smiled when reading Mike Tyler's very nicely observed and honestly expressed Foreword. It resonates with my own discussions with Clarissa and the issues faced by her and, indeed, all the women who have come to me for help. He and I have doubtless discussed many times the issue of what a statistic means to you as an individual. Everyone's perception of risk and benefit is unique, even if we mostly draw similar ultimate conclusions. Understanding this is at the very core of ensuring that we help people make sensible decisions that are right for them.

The principles of inheritance and managing risk are simple and it should be easy to get them right. Many women are identified with BRCA mutation at the right time and their risk is managed appropriately. But in reality many women find it hard to get the right advice and to feel secure that they are making the best decision for them. And of course the point is not just to manage the actual risk of getting a cancer but to reduce the anxiety and distress that naturally surrounds being in a family with any cancer-causing mutation. A technical solution without reassurance and context will only go part way to relieving that distress.

The finer details of how to manage that increased risk are more subtle. They include important issues such as whether and, more importantly, when to have screening or preventive 'risk-reducing' surgery and exactly what surgery to have. For this, as well as having a deep knowledge of the facts, doctors need to spend time exploring those concerns with their patients. More than giving advice and information, or even just recommending tests and operations, doctors need to understand their patients' hopes, fears and beliefs. Patients need to have faith in their surgeons' technical skills of course. But they also need to be confident that their doctors are guiding them in the right direction and understand their worries. Clarissa's journey will give healthcare professionals insight into what all our patients go through.

In my practice, I see women having screening who don't need it and women who should have screening who have been falsely reassured that they don't; women whose family history isn't strong and who aren't at increased risk but whose anxiety is increased by arranging screening they don't need; women with strong family histories who probably are at risk who've started screening tests but have not been offered genetic tests or risk-reducing surgery when it was appropriate; even women denied all access to even simple screening tests. Similarly, people whose family history suggests that there must be a responsible mutation need to be able to manage their risk even if a mutation has not been found.

It is in this that women, and men, carrying BRCA mutations need access to usable and accurate information. In her book, Clarissa has made the most up-to-date evidence and advice available to all. She has gone to great lengths to ensure it is accurate and balanced and I sincerely hope and believe that it will help both carriers and healthcare professionals reduce the physical and psychological burden that BRCA mutations bring to society. It will certainly help those carrying these mutations know what questions they will want to ask their doctors. Bravo, indeed.

Alasdair Drake, Consultant Gynaecologist &
Gynaecological Oncologist

About the author

Clarissa Foster is a qualified Human Biology teacher at FE level and an experienced medical writer. She is also a health blogger and an 'expert patient' in relation to BRCA gene mutations.

To produce this book she has worked with consultant gynaecological oncologist, Alasdair Drake, and consultant plastic and reconstructive surgeon, Michael Tyler.

Understanding BRCA has been highly commended by the British Medical Association in the 2018 BMA Book Awards and Clarissa also received the Beryl Bainbridge First Time Author Award in 2019.

Explanatory note

Throughout the book the author has used scientific terms, explained in plain English on their first appearance. All these terms are listed and explained in the Glossary section starting on page 258.

Acknowledgements

I would like to thank my husband, James, for being there every step of the way, both throughout my journey and during the writing of this book. I love you so much.

Thank you to Mr Alasdair Drake, consultant gynaecologist and gynaecological oncologist at the Spire Harpenden Hospital, England, who performed my salpingo-oophorectomy and who also kindly gave his time and expertise throughout the writing of this book. Thanks also to Mr Michael Tyler, consultant plastic and reconstructive surgeon, and his team, at Stoke Mandeville Hospital, England, who performed my mastectomy and reconstruction and who also kindly gave his time and expertise. I am eternally grateful to you both for what you have done for me; words cannot possibly thank you enough.

Thanks also to Mrs Kashmir Randhawa, genetic counsellor at the Thames Regional Genetics Service in Harrow, Middlesex, England, for answering my many questions and for reviewing the genetic counselling section of this book.

I would like to thank the following people and organisations for their expertise and for reviewing the relevant sections of this book; all help has been greatly appreciated:

- Dr Lisa Walker, consultant in clinical genetics at Oxford University Hospitals NHS Foundation Trust Oxford, England;
- Adam Rosenthal PhD FRCOG, consultant gynaecologist, University College London Hospitals NHS Foundation Trust, for

reviewing the ovarian cancer screening section;
- Dr Mohnish Suri, consultant clinical geneticist at Nottingham Clinical Genetics Service, Nottingham City Hospital, Nottingham, England;
- Mr Tom Walton, consultant urological surgeon at Nottingham University Hospital, Nottingham, England;
- Mr Giles Cunnick, consultant breast and general surgeon, at Wycombe Hospital, High Wycombe, England;
- Dr Emilie Wilkes, consultant hepatologist, Nottingham University Hospitals NHS Trust, City Hospital Campus, Nottingham, England;
- Dr Swarna Magapu, dermatologist, London, England;
- Mr Kian Chin, MB ChB, FRCS (Eng), consultant breast surgeon, Milton Keynes University Hospital Trust, Milton Keynes, England;
- Mr Alan R Taylor FRCS, FRCS(Ed), consultant breast and general surgeon;
- Miss Nicola Petrie, consultant plastic and reconstructive surgeon, John Radcliffe Hospital, Oxford, England;
- Mrs Kathy Abernethy, senior nurse specialist at the Menopause Clinical and Research Unit, Northwick Park Hospital, Harrow, England; and
- The genetics counsellors at the North West Thames Regional Genetics Service in Harrow, Middlesex, England.

I would also like to thank all of the researchers whose studies I have referred to within this book. Thanks also to Cancer Research UK, which has been an invaluable source of information throughout the writing of this book.

Jill Mueller, Helen Silvester-Burnop, Julie Parish and Claire Whittaker, thank you for sharing your own experiences and for showing me that it is possible to one day come out the other side.

Thank you, also, to Dave Pinchbeck, for your tireless efforts proofreading my book; your help has been invaluable.

Acknowledgements

Thank you to Georgina Bentliff of Hammersmith Books for accepting my book for publication. Thank you also to Ravinder Crone of Ravinder Crone Photography, Leighton Buzzard, Bedfordshire, England for the photograph shown on the cover of this book and to Andy Ginger, of Barrett & Coe photography, Leighton Buzzard, Bedfordshire, England, for the portrait image used to promote this book.

Last, but not least, thank you also to Angelina Jolie for so bravely sharing with the world your decision to undergo a mastectomy and the removal of your ovaries; you have shown the world that it is possible to undergo these surgeries and to remain a beautiful woman. I have the greatest respect and admiration for you; thank you for helping me personally to remain positive and strong throughout my own journey.

Source of illustrations

I would like to thank the following people and organisations for permission to use the illustrations within this book: Cancer Research UK for Figures 7, 8, 9, 10 and 11 in Section III: Cancer and its relationship with BRCA gene mutations; Matthew Carter for Figures 1, 2, 4, 12, 13, 14 and 15 throughout this book; the Nottingham Cytogenetics Laboratory for Figure 3 (The human karyotype); and the American College of Radiology for Figure 17 detailing levels of breast density; this comes from the information brochure *Breast Density - Breast cancer screening*. I would also like to thank the Royal Marsden Hospital for the data taken from *A Beginner's Guide to BRCA1 and BRCA2* on which Figure 6 and Tables 1-4 have been based.

Introduction

BRCA (pronounced 'bracka') stands for **BR**east **CA**ncer susceptibility gene. There are two BRCA genes – BRCA1 and BRCA2. These genes function as tumour suppressors, helping to prevent the formation of cancer. When either of these genes carries a mutation, a woman has a high risk of developing breast and ovarian cancer, and men with these mutations are also at increased risk of breast and prostate cancer. Mutations in these genes have also been associated with a small increased risk of several additional types of cancer (see page 92).

At the age of 35, I was found to carry a harmful mutation in the second breast cancer (BRCA2) gene and statistics suggested that I had a 45-85% chance of developing breast cancer and a 10-30% risk of developing ovarian cancer during my lifetime, which is much higher than in the general population (see page 38).

Finding out that you carry a BRCA mutation is hard, and if this happens to you, you will have a great many questions that you will feel desperate to find the answers to. I felt overwhelmed and scared of the future that lay ahead. I desperately wanted to connect with other women who were going through the same thing as me and to find answers to my many questions. I looked for a BRCA support group locally, but there were none. I also looked for a book but none seemed to offer what I was looking for. I was eager to meet with the consultants that I had been referred to, but this process takes time and it was frustrating waiting for these appointments. I hoped they would be able to answer all of my questions but, in reality, even the consultants didn't have all the answers as we do not yet fully understand the BRCA genes and their impact. I felt very frightened, alone and frustrated that there seemed to be so little help and support and I wanted this to change. I decided, therefore, that once I had come through my own journey, I would write a book with the aim of helping others.

This book aims to improve your understanding of BRCA gene mutations and the various ways in which a carrier can manage his/her mutation, including screening, risk-reducing surgery and chemoprevention, with reference to relevant research. In the last part of this book, I share with you my own personal journey of undergoing risk-reducing surgery, including the removal of my ovaries and fallopian tubes (known as a bilateral salpingo-oophorectomy, pronounced oo-for-ek-tuh-mee) and the removal of my breast tissue while retaining my nipples (known as a bilateral, nipple-sparing mastectomy).

I detail, openly and honestly, the emotions I felt before, during and after my surgeries, along with the physical experience of undergoing these operations and the surgically-induced menopause which follows the removal of both ovaries. I will share the effect, if any, that these operations have had on my body image, identity and sexual functioning.

This book aims to answer the many questions that I personally had, including those that you may feel are simply too uncomfortable to ask. I felt anxious about so many things but, having come through my own journey, I realise now that I needn't have worried anywhere near as much as I did. I really wish I had known then what I know now; it would have spared me a lot of fear and anxiety.

If you have been found to carry a BRCA gene mutation, I hope that by sharing my journey with you, you will see for yourself that this journey, albeit very tough, may not be as terrifying and as insurmountable as you may be feeling right now. You will get through this – I did and you can too. And, while I appreciate you may not be feeling this way now, you may even be nicely surprised by the positive ways in which this journey may change you as a person.

I am an Advanced-level Human Biology teacher and have experience of teaching both GCSE and Advanced-level (A-level) Human Biology. I also have experience of medical writing and have drawn from both of these skills throughout the writing of this book.

My desire to help others has inspired me not only to write this book, but also to set up a website to offer my support to women and men worldwide who have been found to carry, or who believe they may carry, a BRCA1 or BRCA2 gene mutation.

Section I

Living with BRCA gene mutations

Before embarking on the 'information' section of this book (Section II, page 15), I begin with a chapter relating to my personal experience of the havoc BRCA gene mutations can wreak so that it is easier to understand why much of the detail in Section II is relevant and why I made the momentous decision I did to have risk-reducing surgery, described in Section V (page 181). If aggressive cancer strikes the relatively young parent of dependant children, the results can be particularly devastating and have repercussions for a great many people down the years. I have also included a chapter about the history of BRCA and which ethnicities and populations are more likely to be living with a BRCA gene mutation.

1.
How it began

In 1995, at the age of 44 years, my mother developed a few symptoms that were unusual, including a bloated abdomen, backache, needing to pass urine more frequently, constipation and general malaise. I was 16 years old at the time and at sixth-form college.

My mum had always been a fit and healthy person and was very rarely ill. She ate a healthy diet, very rarely drank alcohol – her only bad habit was smoking. She had always enjoyed a very slim, petite figure throughout her life. When she developed a swelling in her lower abdomen and didn't feel her normal self, it was clear that something was wrong.

She visited her family doctor on numerous occasions but, sadly, her cancer was missed and a number of months passed before it was finally diagnosed. A blood test was carried out to look for the cancer antigen 125 (CA-125) which is produced by some ovarian cancer cells. The test revealed an elevated CA-125 level of 450 units/ml and, given the presence of a mass, ovarian cancer was strongly suspected.

Within a couple of weeks, she had had a total abdominal hysterectomy with bilateral salpingo-oophorectomy to remove her ovaries, fallopian tubes, womb and cervix. After her surgery, the surgeon explained that he had found a tumour about the size of a small grapefruit on each ovary. There was also evidence that the cancer had spread to the peritoneum – a membrane that lines the abdominal cavity and supports the abdominal organs.

The doctors soon confirmed that she did, indeed, have ovarian cancer and she was diagnosed with advanced stage (stage III/IV) bilateral ovarian cancer with metastases to the peritoneum. Very soon afterwards, she started a course of cisplatin chemotherapy, typically used to treat ovarian cancer.

Seeing my mum endure chemotherapy was really tough. After each chemotherapy session she would be very ill and unable to carry on everyday life. She would spend the next few days in bed, only surfacing to vomit. She also experienced some of the more occasional side-effects, including a metallic taste to her food which, in turn, led to a loss of appetite and subsequent weight loss. She later went on to develop a permanent ringing in her ears (tinnitus), a very common side-effect with cisplatin treatment.

Probably the most upsetting side-effect was watching my mum lose all of her hair, including her eyelashes and eyebrows, within a few weeks of starting chemotherapy. She was a beautiful, proud lady who always took care of her appearance and being a hairdresser by profession made it all the more upsetting. Clumps of her hair started to fall out and, with this, my mum lost confidence in her appearance.

I would spend my breaks from coursework and exam revision sitting on Mum's bed, holding her hand, or stroking her head and just being there for her in whatever way I could. I loved her so much and wanted to do whatever I could to make life more bearable for her. Living through a diagnosis of cancer with someone you love is incredibly tough. I felt very alone and I carried a huge weight of emotion on my shoulders. I kept these emotions to myself, often pretending that I was okay so as to not add to Mum's stress levels but, in reality, I was struggling and terrified of losing her. I didn't turn to friends for support because I felt they couldn't possibly understand what I was going through. I lost any sense of being carefree, often finding it hard to enjoy myself. All the while, I felt overshadowed by the fear of my mum's illness and of one day losing her to cancer. It forced me to grow up very quickly and I often felt more mature than friends around me.

Over the course of my time at college, my mum underwent several courses of chemotherapy as the cancer always returned. I spent many nights during this time unable to sleep, wondering if Mum was going to die and, if so, when this would be. Would she deteriorate suddenly, or would it be gradual? Would she go to bed one night and not awake the next morning? I had no idea – how could I possibly have any idea? I had never seen anyone die before. I decided to visit the nurse at my family doctor's and I asked if she thought she would die. The nurse at the practice said, 'Yes, she is very likely to.' Hearing this wasn't easy but, in my heart, I knew it was true.

I worried a great deal about whether or not to go to university when I turned 18 years old – what if Mum died whilst I was away from home? This thought terrified me. I wondered if I should delay going to university and stay at home so that I could continue to support her until the end. I asked her if she would like me to defer my application but, as any mother would do, she told me to continue with my plans.

There were periods when my mum was given the all clear, and told she was in remission, but the fear of the cancer coming back continued to hang over us all and, sadly, these periods of remission were only ever short-lived. The cancer always came back. My mum never returned to being the same, relatively carefree person that she had been prior to her diagnosis of cancer.

In the summer of 1996, during the revision period for my final set of A-level exams, my mum went out for what I thought was a shopping day with a friend – I was pleased to see her doing something nice for herself. I studied hard that day, as I had always done, and I was looking forward to the end of my exams in a few days' time. Late afternoon, I heard her return home; she popped into my room to see how my revision was going. I immediately noticed that both her arms, and the back of one hand, had cotton wool and tape stuck to them. My heart sank. The cancer was back and she had started yet another course of chemotherapy. I wondered just how much more her little body could handle of this aggressive chemotherapy.

I had been really looking forward to finishing my last exam and enjoying the summer before moving to Loughborough University and, now, I wondered how on earth I would be able to leave my mum. I again considered postponing university but, at the same time, now that it was only round the corner, I wanted to go. I had worked so hard to get to this point and I had been looking forward to starting a life for myself. I tried my hardest to focus on my studies, at least for a few more days until I had finished my exams.

In August, my A-level results were available for collection from my college. I was excited, and nervous, but I was confident that I would have achieved the grades I needed. I opened the envelope as quickly as I could, eager to see my results. I was so pleased to have exceeded the grades required to study Human Biology at the university of my choice. Despite the tremendous strain I had been under throughout my time at college, all of my hard work had paid off.

At the end of September 1996, I left my home and travelled to Loughborough. I was excited about the start of my new life, but it was overshadowed by the worry of leaving my mum. Mum and I arrived at the campus and we were directed to my halls of residence. The room was basic, but perfectly good enough, and I was excited that this would be my home for the next year.

Once I had finished unpacking the time had come to say goodbye, but I didn't feel ready to do so. I felt so much emotion come to the surface but, as always, I held back the tears. I looked into my mum's eyes; neither of us were able to speak. I wondered if this would be the last time I saw her and I could feel that she was asking herself the same thing. Still trying to hold back my tears, I told her I loved her and we cuddled for longer than we had ever done before. Saying goodbye to my mum on that day was one of the hardest things I have ever had to do in my life.

My mum continued to battle with her cancer throughout my first and second years at university, but the more time passed, the more I began to realise that she couldn't fight it forever. Heading home for the Christmas of my second year, I was looking forward to seeing my mum; I had missed her. Sitting on the train heading to London, I couldn't help but feel that this would be her last Christmas. I imagined future Christmases without her and how they wouldn't be the same again. I felt deeply saddened. Christmas Day was overshadowed by this sadness and I could see in my mum's eyes that she knew it would be her last too. I felt close to tears for most of the day, but I tried my best not to dwell on it and instead did my best to make the most of this time with my mum.

In early January, the term restarted and I was soon into my exam period. I continued to have anxiety that mum didn't have long left and, in February, I made the decision to change accommodation to allow me to remain on the campus throughout my final academic year. I knew that if Mum died, our family home would have to be sold, at which point I wouldn't have a home to return to for the holiday periods.

In May, just prior to my final exams, I made a call home, but there was no answer. I knew instinctively that something was very wrong. A while later, I 'phoned home again and this time someone answered. I was told that my mum had been taken into hospital as she was in a lot of pain, but this was all I was told. It was far from the full truth, I knew that, and I realised information was being kept from me because of my exams. I thought about returning home, but I couldn't as my first exam was in a few days' time. I considered informing my department, and delaying my exams, but that seemed more stressful than getting the exams out of the way as soon as possible. I reassured myself that if Mum's death was imminent then, surely, I would be asked to go home. I plodded on with my revision, but it was very hard to concentrate and I found it hard to care about my exams; they seemed so insignificant in the scheme of things. But, at the same time, I knew they were vital to secure the future that I had planned for myself.

My exams came to an end and, in the last couple of days, I took some breathing space to gather my thoughts. I tried to prepare myself for what I knew was coming, but I dreaded the idea of going home to see my mum die. Arriving back home, I headed up the stairs towards my mum's bedroom. I opened the door and saw her sitting up in her bed. She started to cry and described how awful it was to have to tell me that she was dying. My heart sank and I was overcome by the deepest sense of sadness. I was speechless, but yet desperately trying to think of anything to say to make it better. Inside I broke down, but outwardly I wanted to remain strong for my mum. I questioned what good crying would do anyway. I had cried so many tears over the last couple of years and I had reached the point where I was sick of crying.

Shortly after my return home, Mum went back into hospital to help manage her pain. The consultant came and explained to me, in front of my mum, that she was dying and that we needed to start making arrangements. I felt so sorry for Mum having to hear those words yet again and, for me, hearing it from the doctors made it all the more real. Within a few days, the hospital transferred her into a hospice, to make her end as comfortable as possible. She became gradually weaker and weaker.

I had no idea what it would be like to see someone die; I had never seen anything like this before and, of course, this isn't the sort of thing taught at school, or college. I asked the nurses what to expect to help prepare myself. One of them described to me what might happen and I tried to imagine each of the possibilities she'd suggested so that it wouldn't be so frightening when the moment came. I barely slept during this time; I just felt so scared and would only fall asleep as it started to get light outside.

In early August my mum started to deteriorate further, sleeping a lot more in her last few days. I realised that she was beginning to let go and in some ways this brought me comfort knowing the end was near for her sake. On 4th August, I had a particularly strong sense that I needed to go to the hospice and I knew what this meant.

Arriving there, I was immediately met by one of the nurses. She appeared stressed and asked if I had got the message to come as the end was near. The call never arrived, but I had instinctively known anyway.

I walked into Mum's room and I could see she was in a lot of pain – her abdomen was massive. The nurse explained that it had most likely perforated. I felt really helpless; I just wanted it to be over for my mum now – she had been through enough. The nurse came in to give her some more morphine, but it barely seemed to take the edge off the pain.

Around 11 in the evening, it was clear that Mum was de-teriorating further. A doctor came in and checked her pulse. I watched him nervously, frightened by the concern on his face. I felt helpless, and heavy-hearted, just sitting there and waiting for a moment that I had feared so much over the last four years. I asked the doctor if she was okay – silly really when she was far from okay. I asked him if he thought she was going to die soon. 'I'll be surprised if she's still here in the morning,' he responded. I lowered my head and then felt the doctor's comforting hand on my shoulder. I smiled and thanked him for checking on my mum.

Mum continued to go downhill, yet midnight came and went. Out of nowhere, it seemed, I started to panic. I couldn't bear the tension any more. I got up, opened the door and I ran so fast down the stairs that it felt like I was flying. I heard screaming, and realised it was coming from me. Part of me was trying to remain strong and I tried to stop myself, but I couldn't. A nurse came running out of the office and I begged her, 'Please help my mum; please, I'm not ready for her to die!' I realised as I was saying those words that there was nothing that anyone could do to save her, but I was terrified and, even with the years I had had to prepare myself, I still wasn't ready for this moment.

The nurse held me and said she couldn't do anything more, but I didn't want to be held. I wanted to run. I wanted to run out of the hospice and far away from everything. I ran from the nurse and headed for the front door, but somehow, I forced myself to stop, realising that, if I missed Mum's last moments, I would regret it for the rest of my life. I forced myself back up the stairs and again sat down in the chair. My heart was racing faster and harder than it had ever done before. Only moments later, she lapsed into the final stages. Her breathing became shallower and I watched her take her last breath. I remember looking so closely, willing her to breathe again, but she didn't. I remember saying, 'She has gone.' I looked at the clock: it was 12.50 am on the 5th August 1998.

Again I panicked and flew back down the stairs screaming. The nurse came running out, this time realising that my mum had died. She tried to comfort me, but I couldn't bear to be touched. I felt consumed by grief and had the most awful feeling in my chest and stomach that words can't even begin to describe.

After a while, I managed to calm myself down. For my mum's sake, I felt pleased that it was all over but I knew that, for me, it wasn't. I would now have to go through the long process of grieving and living the rest of my life without my mum. I was only 20 years old and life just wasn't fair.

I thought about how I would never hear my mum's voice again, or speak to her on the 'phone. She wouldn't see me turn 21 in a few months' time, nor would she see me graduate. I thought also about how she would never meet my future husband, or be there on my wedding day, or see her grandchildren. Our family home would have to be sold and my dog whom I adored would have to be re-homed. I was losing everything I cared about and every ounce of security that I had. I was heart-broken, deeply saddened and very frightened of the future that lay ahead. I was terrified at the prospect of returning to Loughborough in a couple of weeks' time to finish the final year of my degree. I felt that my life was completely unbearable and what I had ahead of me insurmountable.

After the funeral I travelled back to Loughborough to finish my third, and final, year, but I really didn't know if I had the strength to get through it. I had nothing left in me but, at the same time, I knew that any bit of strength I could find would be directed towards my degree and towards making a great future for myself.

During that final year, I studied the Genetics of Cancer and I read about the first and second breast cancer genes (BRCA1 and BRCA2). I became aware that harmful mutations in these genes mean that a woman has a high risk of breast and ovarian cancer, and men with these mutations are also at increased risk of breast cancer and prostate cancer. Mutations in these genes have also been associated with small increased risks of several additional types of cancer.

I learnt that these mutations were common in people with Ashkenazi Jewish ancestry and I reflected on my mum saying that her father was Jewish, and that his family had originated from Eastern Europe. Bearing this and my mum's diagnosis with ovarian cancer at an early age in mind, I suspected that there was a strong possibility that she had carried a BRCA gene mutation. If so, then I would have a 50:50 chance of carrying it too. For now though, I needed to put this possibility to the back of my mind and concentrate on finishing my degree.

In the summer of 1999, I finished the final exam of my degree. I felt incredibly pleased with myself for getting through it and in

July I graduated with a BSc (Hons.) in Human Biology. I enjoyed the day as much as I could, but it was overshadowed by the sadness of my mum not being there. Walking up on to the stage with a beaming smile on my face, heading towards my head of department to collect my certificate, I felt immensely proud of what I had achieved. He shook my hand and said, 'Well done, Clarissa, you have done so well!' I knew what he meant and that was a very special moment for me.

After graduation, and with our family home having been sold, I decided to set up home in Loughborough, for a while at least, until I knew what I wanted for my future. I rented a room in a house and met my husband-to-be, James, who was a student at the university. I found a lot of happiness and security around this time and my life really started to take off. I studied for a Postgraduate Certificate in Education (PGCE) and when our studies were completed, James and I were able to start planning our wedding. We married in 2005 and I gave birth to our first baby, Isabelle, in 2007. I was blown away by the depth of love that I felt for her. Becoming a mum made me appreciate just how much my mum must have loved me. I felt a deep sadness that she couldn't be there to enjoy her granddaughter and it was hard for me to not have her help and support at this point in my life.

In February 2010, I gave birth to our second child, Ben. I adored him just as much as his sister and, with his arrival, our beautiful family felt complete.

Since becoming a mum, I have realised more than ever the importance of being around for my children and being able to see them grow up. The thought of them living through what I experienced with my mum fills me with dread; I was determined I would do anything I possibly could to avoid that and to ensure that I would be there for them for as long as possible. I decided to talk with my family doctor about the possibility of my mother having carried a BRCA gene mutation; she held the opinion that it was very unlikely, seeing as she was the only family member to have presented with ovarian cancer and given that there are, to the best of my knowledge, no cases of breast cancer within our family. My family doctor explained that, under the current National Institute for Clinical Excellence (NICE) guidelines, I was not eligible for referral for BRCA gene mutation testing under the NHS.

That all changed when, towards the end of 2012, when I was 34 years old, I learned that my older sister had pursued private testing in the US and been found to carry a harmful BRCA2 mutation. This confirmed beyond any reasonable doubt that my mum must have also carried this mutation and, if so, then I would have a 50:50 chance of being a carrier also. I was now eligible under the NICE guidelines for referral to a genetic counsellor for BRCA gene testing.

On my 35th birthday, in February 2013, I attended an initial appointment with a genetic counsellor to discuss the possibility of being tested. I explained my reasons for doing this and, at the end of this first meeting, a blood sample was taken. Four weeks later, in March 2013, I was informed that I carried a harmful BRCA2 gene mutation. Finding out that I carried this mutation wasn't the news that I had hoped for but, at the same time, it didn't come as a surprise. It was, however, alarming to be told that I had a much greater risk of developing breast and ovarian cancer than people in the general population,[1] as well as a small increased risk of several additional types of cancer.

I was in a state of shock and I feared that I would die in the same way that I had seen my mum do. I feared also for my children and their future health. I wondered whether this mutation had been passed down to them, and I found myself imagining them being diagnosed with cancer. The thought of this was just too much to bear and it was, by far, the most distressing of my emotions. However, I reminded myself that, for now at least, I had to put the worry of my children's future to one side until they themselves were old enough to be tested.

The most important thing for now was coming to terms with my news and making a decision about how I would lower my risk of developing breast and ovarian cancer. I felt determined to spare my children the trauma of seeing their mother live through cancer and to improve the likelihood that I would be around to support them in the future.

On a positive note, I felt incredibly lucky to know that I carried a harmful BRCA mutation before cancer had struck and to be empowered to take action to lower my risk of developing cancer. Sadly, this isn't often an option for women who only learn of their mutation after cancer has been diagnosed. I trusted that, no matter how tough my own journey would be, it would be easier than living through cancer. Reminding myself of this fact is ultimately what helped to give me the strength, focus and determination to get through my own journey, to which I will return in the final section of this book. Before I continue with my personal story I want to share with you everything I have learnt about the BRCA genes and their relationship with cancer, and what the implications of this are for one's future health.

2.
The history of BRCA

In 1994, Dr Mark Skolnick and his colleagues at Myriad Genetics in the USA announced that they had identified the first breast cancer gene (BRCA1). This effectively put an end to a five-year competition that had been raging among several research groups in North America and Europe.[2] The following year a second breast cancer gene (BRCA2) was discovered in England by Professor Michael Stratton and Dr Richard Wooster at the Institute of Cancer Research. Since this time, many hundreds of mutations have been identified and the search for more continues.

The BRCA genes are extremely large and identifying a cancer-causing mutation is like finding a needle in a haystack. However, more than 1600 mutations have been identified in BRCA1, and more than 1800 in BRCA2.[3]

The exact number of people affected by BRCA gene mutations is unknown. However, in the UK, it is predicted that the faulty BRCA genes occur in around one in every 400 people, but as many as one in 40 people of Ashkenazi Jewish (Eastern Europe) origin may carry a faulty gene.[4] In the United States, about one in every 500 women carries either a BRCA1 or BRCA2 gene mutation.[5] More specifically, according to the American Congress of Obstetricians and Gynaecologists (ACOG), about one in 300 people carries a BRCA1 mutation and one in 800 carries a BRCA2 mutation.[6] However, it is nearly impossible to know precisely how common these mutations are within any population. Only by testing everyone in the population would we be able to calculate how common these mutations are, but this would prove too costly.

Ashkenazi Jews and BRCA

Approximately 29 generations, or 3000 years, ago, an ancestor of Eastern European Jews developed a defect in the DNA coding for the BRCA2 gene. This DNA defect, known as the 6174delT mutation, has since been passed from generation to generation.

Ashkenazi Jews are the Jews of France, Germany and Eastern Europe and their descendants. Approximately 80% of the Jews in the world today are Ashkenazim, with the remainder primarily Sephardic. Although Ashkenazi Jews are found around the world, for many centuries they were a geographically isolated population and their ancestry can be traced back to a small number of members known as 'founders'. They lived in the medieval era, about 600 to 800 years ago, and numbered just 350 or so people. Because the Ashkenazi community started out so small, and remained genetically isolated, it developed a higher number of disease-causing mutations, such as BRCA1 and BRCA2 gene mutations which confer high risks of breast and ovarian cancer. Over time, the genetic traits of these early Ashkenazi 'founders' have been passed down through generations.

In particular, there are three mutations that account for the majority of the BRCA mutations seen in persons of Ashkenazi Jewish ancestry: two common mutations in the BRCA1 gene (185delAG and 5382insC) and one common mutation in BRCA2 (6174delT). Over 2% of Ashkenazi Jews carry one of these three founder mutations.[7]

Although BRCA gene mutations are more common in Jewish people of Ashkenazi origin, they are also frequently found in French Canadian, Icelandic and Finnish backgrounds, but they can occur in anyone. It is important to bear in mind that although the founder mutations originate in Ashkenazim, the mixing of Jews within Europe means that Sephardic Jews cannot assume that they are not at increased risk of also carrying a BRCA gene mutation.

Certain mutations are most commonly found within specific ethnic groups. For example, BRCA1 (5382insC, C61G and 4153delA) is commonly found in people with Polish ancestry, BRCA1 (2804delAA) in Dutch, BRCA1 (1081delG) in Chinese, BRCA1 (4153delA, 5382insC) in Russian and BRCA1 (1832del5, 5296del4) in African-American groups.[7] For a more comprehensive list of the most common and founder mutations found in European populations, please see the Appendix, page 277.

Section II

Understanding BRCA gene mutations

In this section of the book I present all the information I would like to have had access to when I was found to be a BRCA gene mutation carrier and had to make decisions about managing the associated risks. I very much hope you will find it useful at a time in your life when sound knowledge can make an important difference.

My purpose, in gathering together here all my findings, is to save other carriers, and their families and friends, the lengthy task of researching BRCA all over again.

3.
What is the BRCA gene?

This section of the book aims to provide an easy-to-understand explanation of the science relating to the BRCA gene, its role within our body and what it means if this gene carries a harmful mutation. To gain this understanding, we need first to look at basic cell structure, including the nucleus, chromosomes, genes, DNA and their role in cell division. We need to consider changes in the DNA known as mutations which, if harmful, can lead to diseases such as cancer. We will look at the different types of BRCA mutations (e.g. deletion mutations) that may occur, and explain how BRCA gene mutations are inherited from our parents. This section will also examine who is most at risk of carrying BRCA gene mutations and what their risk of developing cancer is, compared with women who do not carry a mutation.

Also included in this section is a BRCA statistics table, produced by the Royal Marsden Hospital, London, England, which details the percentage risks for breast cancer for both men and women, ovarian cancer and prostate cancer for both BRCA1 and BRCA2 mutation carriers; it also details the effect of age on the risk of developing breast cancer.

Finally, this section explores the common misconceptions people have about the BRCA genes and the possible evolutionary advantages or benefits of carrying a BRCA gene mutation. Genes which are harmful and provide no benefit at all will be naturally removed from the gene pool, but it's important to note that mutated BRCA genes are continuing within the gene pool and, for this reason, these mutations are likely to be beneficial as well.

Note: This chapter starts with the absolute basics of cell biology. Although you may already be familiar with this, it is, where possible, BRCA-specific and much of this will aid your understanding of later sections of this book.

A cell

As you probably already know, a cell is the basic functioning unit in a living organism. An adult human body is made up of about 37 trillion cells, all working together to create a highly organised and sophisticated living organism. The most prominent feature of a cell is the nucleus and its function is to control the cell's activity and cell division. The nucleus contains the genetic material (the DNA) in the form of chromosomes, which we will look at shortly.

Our body contains several hundred different types of specialised cells. These different types of cells are specifically suited to the function that they perform.

Every cell in the body contains the same set of genes, which provides a library of instructions for everything the cell could possibly do. However, not all the genes in a cell are switched on ('expressed') and it is this that gives each individual type of cell its own unique specialisation. For example, a heart cell still contains all the same genes as a liver cell, but only the genes associated with heart cell properties need to be switched on. The genes that are switched on can then be used by the cell as a template for producing proteins. By turning genes on and off, the cell can make sure that the right proteins are made at the right time in the right cells. For example, the BRCA1 and BRCA2 genes that are turned on, or 'expressed', within the breast cells will be used as a template for producing a tumour suppressor protein which helps to prevent the formation of a breast tumour. However, the BRCA genes are housekeeping genes as they are, in fact, expressed within every cell of the body and not only in breast and ovarian cells.

Chromosomes

A chromosome is a rod-like structure present in the nucleus of nearly every cell in the body. The only exceptions are the red blood cells which do not have a nucleus, which allows for more space for oxygen to be transported around the body.

Chromosomes are made up of long strands of DNA within the nucleus of the cell and they contain an enormous number of genes. If the DNA in one cell was stretched all the way out, it would be about 2 metres long and if we stretched out the DNA in all your cells put together, it would be able to wrap around the Earth's equator 2.5 million times, or about twice the diameter of our solar system.

Each chromosome has a constriction point called the centromere, which divides the chromosome into two sections or 'arms'. The p arms are the short arms and the q arms are the long arms (see Figure 1).

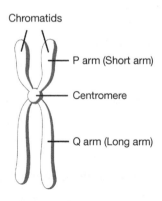

Figure 1: A single chromosome

Most human cells have 23 pairs of chromosomes – or 46 chromosomes in total. Each cell contains two sets of chromosomes – one set from your mother and the other from your father.

In Figure 2, there is a cell with a cell nucleus, within which there are 23 pairs of chromosomes. Each chromosome is made up of DNA tightly coiled many times and along the DNA, there are genes.

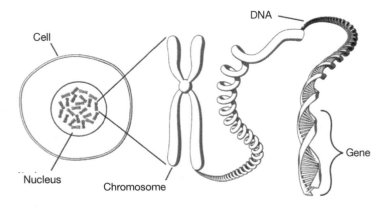

Figure 2: Diagram of DNA and how it is incorporated in a cell

It is possible to take a picture of the chromosomes from within one of our cells and arrange them depending on their size. This is known as a 'human karyotype' and may be seen in Figure 3.

Two chromosomes, known as the sex chromosomes, specify gender (XX for female and XY for male). The rest are arranged in pairs, numbered 1 to 22, from largest to smallest, and they are known as 'autosomes'. This arrangement helps scientists quickly identify chromosomal alterations that may result in a genetic disorder. Most cases of Down syndrome, for example, result from 'trisomy 21', which means each cell in the body has three copies of chromosome 21 instead of the usual two copies. The BRCA1 gene is located on the long (q) arm of chromosome 17 and the BRCA2 gene, which is a larger gene than BRCA1, is found on the long (q) arm of chromosome 13.

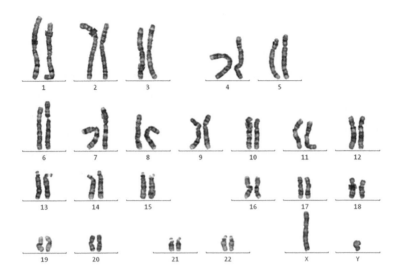

Figure 3: The human karyotype[1]

DNA (deoxyribonucleic acid)

DNA determines certain characteristics (genetic traits) that are passed from parents to children, such as hair colour, eye colour, blood type and the risk of developing certain diseases.

DNA is a long molecule that contains our unique genetic code. Like a recipe book it holds the instructions for making all the proteins which are needed to build and maintain the human body. The information in DNA is stored as a code made up of four different chemical bases: adenine (A), guanine (G), cytosine (C) and thymine (T). Human DNA consists of about three billion bases, and more than 99% of those bases are the same in all people. In humans, a copy of the entire genome – more than three billion DNA base pairs – is contained in all cells that have a nucleus. Our complete set of DNA, including all of our genes, is referred to as the 'human genome'. The order, or sequence, of these bases determines the information available for building and maintaining our bodies, similar to the way in which letters of the alphabet appear in a certain order to form words and sentences.

DNA bases pair up with each other, A with T and C with G, to form units called base pairs. Each base is also attached to a sugar molecule and a phosphate molecule to form a nucleotide. The nucleotides are arranged in two long strands that form a spiral, or 'double helix', as can be seen in Figure 4. The phosphate and the sugar form the 'sugar phosphate backbone' of the DNA helix and the base pairs adenine-thymine and cytosine-guanine form the rungs of the DNA helix.

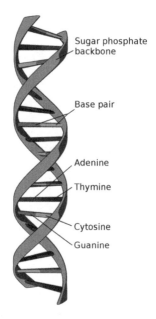

Figure 4: DNA is a double helix formed by base pairs attached to a sugar-phosphate backbone.

An important property of DNA is that it can replicate (make copies of) itself. This is critical when cells divide because each new cell needs to have an exact copy of the DNA present in the old cell.

Cell division

It is important for cells to divide for growth and repair of the body, but it is also important for cells to stop dividing at the right time. If a cell cannot stop dividing when it is supposed to, this can lead to cancer.

Some cells, like skin cells, are constantly dividing to replace the 30,000-40,000 we lose every minute, or around 50 million cells every day. Clearly, this is a lot of skin cells to replace, making cell division in the skin cells particularly important. Other tissues, such as nerve and brain cells, divide much less often.

In cell division, the cell that is dividing is called the 'parent cell' and this divides into two genetically identical 'daughter cells'. Before a cell can divide it needs to replicate its DNA, so that the daughter cells produced contain the same genetic information. This process of cell division is known as 'mitosis'. The normal process of cell division is essential for life; however, if it were to become out of control, cells would continue to divide without stopping and it is this fault that gives rise to tumours.

Genes

Genes are the parts of the body that pass hereditary traits down through families. A gene is any section along the DNA that carries instructions which allow a cell to produce proteins which help our bodies grow and function normally.

Every living being has genes. In humans, genes vary in size from a few hundred DNA bases to more than two million, and the Human Genome Project has estimated that humans have between 20,000 and 25,000 genes in nearly every cell in the body.[2]

Every person has two copies of each gene, one inherited from each parent. Many genes are the same in all people, but some genes are slightly different between people – this is what makes each of us unique. It is our genes that decide whether someone is tall or short, the colour of their hair, the colour of their skin, whether they are more likely to develop certain diseases, whether they are naturally good at sports, and what they look like, to name but a few.

As I have said, a gene consists of a long combination of four different bases, A, G, C and T. Different combinations of these letters (bases) give people different characteristics. For example, a person with the following combination – AACCCGGGGTTT – may have green eyes, while somebody whose combination is – AACCCGGGGTCC – may have blue eyes. In reality, however, these codes would be much longer.

Mutations

A mutation is a permanent change in the DNA sequence of a gene. Sometimes mutations can be useful (for example, mutations in the CcR5 gene can protect individuals against certain strains of HIV) but, more often than not, mutations are harmful because changes in the DNA can change the way a cell behaves. Because genes provide a set of instructions necessary for a cell to work properly, if some of these instructions are damaged by mutation the cell may lose its ability to function properly.

However, mutations are essential for the process of evolution – the change in heritable traits over successive generations. Without mutations, evolution could not occur. Every single human trait – green eyes, red hair, sickle cell-anaemia, a second toe longer than the big toe, and so on – is the result of a genetic mutation somewhere back down the line. Traits may be as innocuous as eye colour or as serious as an increased tendency toward a particular disease, but, in many cases, mutations which are harmful in one way have also been found to be beneficial in another. A good example of this are the genes associated with sickle-cell anaemia, a life-threatening and lifelong disease which affects the ability of the red blood cells to carry oxygen around the body. A person will only be affected by the disease if both copies of the inherited gene are mutated. However, a person with a single mutated gene benefits from being highly protected against malaria, thus explaining the high prevalence of this mutation in geographical areas where malaria is endemic. Therefore, in areas where malaria is a problem, people's chances of survival actually increase if they carry the sickle-cell trait.

Somatic or germline

Mutations can be either 'somatic' or 'germline'. Germline mutations are those which are present in the DNA of sperm or egg cells and it is these mutations which can be passed down from one generation to the next. BRCA mutations that are inherited from our parents are classified as germline, or hereditary, mutations.

When an egg and sperm cell unite, the fertilised egg cell contains DNA from both parents. If this DNA includes a mutation, the child that grows from the fertilised egg will have the mutation in each of his or her cells. The vast majority of BRCA gene mutations will be germline mutations and any cancer which arises from these mutations is referred to as a hereditary cancer.

Somatic (or acquired) mutations are those which arise in any cell in the body that is not a sperm or egg cell. These mutations can only be passed on through cell division within the body in which they arise, and cannot be passed on to the next generation. During the process of cell division, the DNA may not be copied correctly; hence, the daughter cell will not be genetically identical to the parent cell and will instead carry a mutation. If this mistake occurs within the DNA of the BRCA gene, then a harmful mutation may arise within this gene. Rapid growth of the breast epithelial tissue during puberty and pregnancy offers an ideal opportunity for such somatic mutations in the BRCA genes to arise. It is possible, therefore, that an individual may carry a harmful BRCA1 or BRCA2 mutation that was not inherited from either parent, but which arose spontaneously within their own DNA. This BRCA gene mutation would not be present in every cell of the body, as would be true for germline mutations. Having a single mutation alone may not lead to cancer, but accumulated mutations over a period of time are what may eventually lead to cancer.

In other cases, a somatic BRCA mutation occurs in the fertilised egg shortly after the egg and sperm cells unite. As the fertilised egg divides, each resulting cell in the growing embryo will have the mutation. This child will carry a mutation in every cell in the body, but the parents do not and, in this case, there would be no family history of BRCA-associated cancer.

Somatic mutations can also be acquired depending on the environment in which a person lives, as some environmental agents can damage the DNA. For example, radiation released during the nuclear disasters that occurred at Windscale and Chernobyl nuclear power plants, is still affecting, and causing mutations in, the genetic make-up of the people living in those areas. Nearly 30 years after the accident, exposure to iodine-131, a radioactive isotope, may be responsible for thyroid cancers that are still occurring among people who lived in the Chernobyl area and were children or adolescents at the time of the accident.

Cancers which arise as a result of somatic mutations are often referred to as sporadic cancers. A sporadic cancer is one that occurs in people who do not have a family history of that cancer and who also do not have an inherited change in their DNA which would increase their risk for that cancer.

Types of mutation

There are a number of specific types of mutation which can occur. A gene can mutate when, for example, its DNA adds, deletes or substitutes nucleotides. If you have been found to carry a

BRCA gene mutation, you may wish at this point to refer to your results, as this following section will help to clarify what type of mutation you have been found to carry.

Substitution mutations

Substitution mutations (missense mutations) occur when there is an exchange between two bases (i.e. a change in a single 'chemical letter' such as switching an A to a G). This type of mutation results in the substitution of the wrong amino acid in the protein. This can cause an incomplete protein which, in turn, can seriously affect the protein's structure and its ability to function normally. Substitution mutations are indicated by '>'. The BRCA1 mutations c.4808C>G, c.5214C>T, c.5236G>A, c.5460G>T and c.5622C>T are examples of substitution mutations in which one chemical letter is substituted for another.

Insertion mutations

An insertion (or duplication) mutation changes the number of DNA bases in a gene by adding an extra piece of DNA. As a result, the protein made by the gene may not function properly. The number of base pairs inserted can range from only one base pair to thousands. Insertion mutations are indicated by 'ins'. The common founder mutation BRCA1 5382**ins**C is an insertion mutation which occurs when a cytosine (C) base is inserted in position 5382. This may also be written as 5382dupC.

Deletion mutations

Deletions are mutations in which a section of DNA is lost or deleted. As a result, the protein made by the gene is unlikely to function properly. The number of base pairs deleted can again range from one to thousands.

Insertion and deletion mutations are often together dubbed

as 'INDELS' and are usually more harmful than a substitution in which only a single amino acid is altered. Furthermore, deletion mutations might be more harmful than insertions because the deleted fragment of the gene will never be replaced, whereas there could be a possibility of the inserted fragment being released from the mutated gene, in which case the gene would be functional again.[3]

Deletion mutations are indicated by 'del'. Alternatively, where several bases have been inserted or deleted, a number may follow 'ins' or 'del', indicating the number of affected bases. The BRCA1 mutation 185**del**AG is an example of a deletion mutation in which an adenine (A) and a guanine (G) are deleted in nucleotide position 185. The BRCA2 mutation that I have personally been found to carry – c.5130_5133**del**TGTA (5358del4) – is a deletion mutation in which thymine (T), guanine (G), thymine (T) and adenine (A) are deleted in nucleotide position 5130_5133. Another example is the BRCA2 mutation 6174**del**T in which a thymine (T) at nucleotide position 6174 has been deleted.

Deletion and insertion mutations that shift the way the DNA sequence is read are known as frameshift mutations. Insertions and deletions in the DNA can completely change a gene so its message cannot be read correctly. This usually gives rise to a truncated (shortened) protein which cannot function properly.

How BRCA mutations are inherited

As previously mentioned, all of our genes are in pairs, one inherited from each parent. We have inherited one copy of the BRCA1 gene from our mother and one from our father. The same applies to the BRCA2 gene. BRCA mutations can be passed to you from your mother or father.

BRCA mutations are inherited in an 'autosomal dominant' pattern, which means that a single copy of the mutated BRCA1 or BRCA2 gene in each cell is enough to increase the probability of developing certain cancers. When a person with a BRCA mutation has children they may pass along a copy of their normal gene or a copy of the gene with the mutation. Therefore, each child has a 50% chance of inheriting the BRCA mutation and a 50% chance of inheriting the working BRCA gene copy, as is shown in Figure 5.

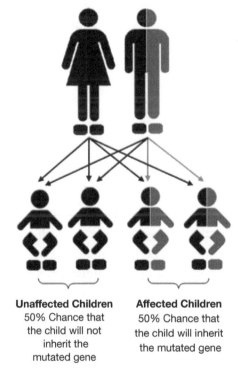

Unaffected Children
50% Chance that
the child will not
inherit the
mutated gene

Affected Children
50% Chance that
the child will inherit
the mutated gene

Figure 5: Autosomal dominant inheritance. There is a 50% chance a child will inherit the mutated gene

This is true for each pregnancy. Each child's risk of carrying the mutation does not depend on whether their sibling has the mutation. However, children who do not inherit the abnormal gene will not be carriers of the mutation and cannot, therefore, pass it on to the next generation. Furthermore, their risk of developing cancer will be the same as that of an individual in the general population. However, children who inherit a BRCA mutation are at an increased risk of developing BRCA-associated cancer and they may also pass the gene mutation on to their children.

Those who inherit a BRCA gene mutation are typically reported as being 'heterozygous' for the familial mutation. This means that an individual has inherited two different versions of a gene, one that is a mutated copy of the gene from one parent, and a normal copy from the other parent.

It is possible, although rare, for both parents to carry a BRCA2 mutation and for a child to inherit two mutated genes. Such individuals are then described as being 'homozygous' for the BRCA2 gene mutation. The BRCA2 gene belongs to a family of genes called FANC (Fanconi anaemia, complementation groups) and inheriting two BRCA2 mutations causes Fanconi anaemia – a very rare, life-threatening, inherited blood disorder that leads to bone marrow failure.

On the other hand, inheriting two BRCA1 mutations (one from each parent) has conventionally been believed to be a lethal birth defect. However, the first confirmed report of a patient harbouring two harmful BRCA1 mutations has been reported in the medical literature. This study, reported in 2013, describes a developmentally delayed patient with short stature and an ovarian cancer diagnosed at 28 years of age, an unusual age even for a BRCA1 mutation carrier. This individual was found to have one gene with a known harmful mutation in BRCA1 (c.2457delC) and a second mutated BRCA1 gene (c.5207T>C), the effects of which are not fully understood.[4] In 2016, a further case of an individual harbouring two BRCA1 mutations was reported. In this study, a 30-year-old woman, with no developmental delay, who developed breast cancer was found to carry a mutation in one BRCA1 gene (c.2681_2682delAA) and another (c.594-2A>C) in the other BRCA1 gene.[5]

It is also possible, although very rare, for one parent to carry a BRCA1 gene mutation and the other a BRCA2 gene mutation, in which case the child will have a 75% likelihood of inheriting one or both of those mutations. In these individuals, the BRCA1 mutation appears to mask the effect of the BRCA2 mutation. As a result, a woman with both mutations has the same risk of breast cancer as a woman with just a BRCA1 mutation.[6] Anecdotal observations (casual observations rather than rigorous scientific analysis) suggest that such women are found to have more frequent and earlier cancers than women with single mutations, but the number of such women identified has been too small for definitive studies.

4.
The effect of BRCA gene mutations

As previously mentioned, every human being has BRCA genes. Healthy BRCA genes – without mutations – function as tumour suppressors. More specifically, BRCA1 and BRCA2 produce tumour suppressor proteins which function to prevent the formation of cancer. These proteins help repair damaged DNA and, therefore, play a part in ensuring the stability of the cell's genetic material.

BRCA genes play a critical part in regulating when cells are allowed to divide and increase in number. When DNA damage is detected in a cell, these genes can stop the cell from multiplying until the damage is repaired. When either of these genes is mutated, or altered, the protein that would normally be produced is absent, or altered, and doesn't function as it should. Often, the protein is truncated (shortened) which prevents it from carrying out its normal function in the cell. As a result, the defective or missing BRCA protein is unable to help repair damaged DNA or fix mutations that occur in other genes. The cells with DNA damage continue to divide and can accumulate further DNA damage that may eventually lead to cancer.

Together, BRCA1 and BRCA2 mutations account for about 20-25% of hereditary breast cancers[7] and 3-5% of all breast cancers.[8] The other 95-97% may occur as a result of other genetic mutations, such as mutations in the TP53 or PALB2 gene, or as a result of environmental factors, including obesity, a poor diet containing too much processed food and a lack of exercise. In addition, BRCA1 and BRCA2 mutations are thought to account for approximately 5-15% of all ovarian cancer cases.[9]

The BRCA mutation itself does not cause cancer to occur and, indeed, some people who carry a BRCA gene mutation may not develop cancer in their lifetime; however, it does mean that carriers of a harmful mutation are at a much greater risk of developing cancer because their cells' ability to repair DNA damage may be impaired by their mutation. It is the accumulation of DNA damage over a period of time which causes a healthy cell to change into a cancerous one.

In a single cell, somewhere in a woman's breast, control over cell division may vanish and the cell begins to divide and increase rapidly in number. The cell continues to divide when it should not, again and again, resulting in the formation of a tumour. When the growth consists of millions of cells, the woman may notice a lump or puckering in the skin of her breast, which may be detected by a magnetic resonance imaging (MRI) scan or by mammography.

Why is it that breast and ovarian cancers are disproportionately high in BRCA mutation carriers?

Scientists are yet to be certain of why these cancers are disproportionately high in BRCA mutation carriers. However, one possibility is that sex hormone imbalance and an altered sensitivity of the breasts and ovaries to oestrogen and progesterone might explain why such women have a disproportionately high risk of developing breast and ovarian cancer. A study published in 2013 which sought to identify differences in hormone regulation between BRCA1/2 mutation carriers and women without BRCA gene mutations found that women with BRCA1/2 gene mutations had higher levels of oestrogen and progesterone, known risk factors for breast cancer. According to the study, higher levels of oestrogen in mutation carriers are also compatible with this hormone having a role in the development of ovarian cancer.[10]

Who is at risk of having a BRCA mutation?

A person may be at increased risk of having a mutation if their family history includes any of the following:

- multiple relatives with breast cancer;
- any relatives with ovarian cancer;
- relatives diagnosed with breast cancer before age 50;
- a relative with cancer in both breasts;
- a relative with both breast and ovarian cancers;
- a male relative with breast cancer;
- Ashkenazi Jewish ancestry (Central or Eastern European), and a relative with breast or ovarian cancer;
- a relative with a known BRCA gene mutation.

If none of these family history patterns fits, there is a low probability of an individual having a BRCA1 or BRCA2 mutation.

Having a strong family tendency towards breast and/or ovarian cancer may suggest the presence of 'hereditary breast and ovarian cancer syndrome' (HBOC), an inherited disorder that increases a person's risk of getting breast cancer and ovarian cancer. BRCA gene mutations are responsible for the majority of hereditary breast and ovarian cancers. However, a family may have several individuals with breast cancer but no indication of a harmful BRCA1 or BRCA2 mutation. Multiple cases of the same cancers within a family strongly suggest a family inheritance pattern, but this may be due to mutations in other genes besides the BRCA gene. There is ongoing research, known as the Breast and Ovarian Cancer Susceptibility (BOCS) study, which is looking for other genes that may be responsible for the increased risk of breast and ovarian cancer in some families. For more information about this study, please see the 'Websites for further information' section (page 304) or contact a genetic counsellor. In addition, some centres in the UK are running multi-gene panel testing in BRCA-negative families with a very strong history of breast or ovarian cancer, and mutations in other genes have been found in these families.

What is a BRCA mutation carrier's risk compared with other women?

Women in the UK have a one in eight or 12.5% chance, on average, of developing breast cancer in their lifetime. Women with one or two close relatives affected with breast cancer have a lifetime risk of 17-30%, depending on the specific family history. Women who have a BRCA1 gene mutation have a 60-90% lifetime risk and women who have a BRCA2 gene mutation have a 45-85% lifetime risk.[11] Also, BRCA mutation carriers have a high chance that cancer will occur bilaterally – that is, that the cancer will arise in both breasts or in both ovaries.[12]

Approximately 2% of women in the general population will develop ovarian cancer.[13] However, women who have a BRCA1 gene mutation have a 40-60% lifetime risk of developing ovarian cancer, and women with the faulty BRCA2 gene have a 10-30% lifetime risk. Because different studies look at different populations, and because different types of mutations have somewhat different risks, the risk is best expressed as a range, rather than a single number, as may be seen in Table 1.

Table 1: Lifetime risk of breast and ovarian cancer in women with and without BRCA gene mutations

Type of cancer	Risk for the general population, UK	Risk with BRCA1 mutation	Risk with BRCA2 mutation
Breast	12.5%	60-90%	45-85%
Ovary	2%	40-60%	10-30%

Data only taken from The Royal Marsden's *A Beginner's Guide to BRCA1 and BRCA2*[11]

In BRCA mutation carriers, these cancers characteristically occur before the age of 50. However, it is important to remember that not everyone who carries a BRCA gene mutation will go on to develop cancer. The reason for this can be explained by the concept of 'penetrance'. Penetrance refers to the proportion of people with a particular genetic change, such as a mutation, who go on to develop the associated disease. A condition is said to show 100% penetrance if symptoms are present in all individuals who have the disease-causing mutation. However, if some people with a particular mutation do not develop the disorder, the condition is said to have reduced or incomplete penetrance. Familial breast cancer due to mutations in the BRCA1 or BRCA2 genes is an example of a condition which shows incomplete penetrance – not everyone who carries a mutation will go on to develop cancer. In other words, carrying a BRCA mutation does not confer a 100% risk for disease.

Females with a mutation in the BRCA1 gene have up to a 90% lifetime risk of developing breast cancer. The penetrance is therefore 90% (90 people out of a 100) – of those with the mutation, 90% will develop the disease, while 10% (10 people) will not.

Doctors cannot predict which people with these mutations will develop cancer, or when the tumours will develop. This incomplete penetrance probably results from a combination of genetic, environmental and lifestyle factors, many of which are unknown. This phenomenon can make it challenging for genetics professionals to interpret a person's family medical history and predict the likelihood of mutation carriers developing cancer. Because of this, individuals who have been found to carry a mutation are informed that their risk of developing cancer lies somewhere within a given range, rather than a single number.

The Royal Marsden Hospital has produced a very informative table (see Table 2) to show the cancer risks for female BRCA mutation carriers.

Table 2: Cancer risks associated with BRCA1/2

	BRCA1	BRCA2
Breast cancer, in unaffected women (up to age 80)	60–90%	45–85%
Women with breast cancer (in one breast). Lifetime risk of a new cancer in the other breast	50% (5 year risk of new breast cancer ~10%)	50% (5 year risk of new breast cancer ~ 5–10%)
Ovarian cancer, lifetime risk	40–60% Risk increases from age 40	10–30% Risk increases from mid 40s

The Royal Marsden's *A Beginner's Guide to BRCA1 and BRCA2*[11]

We can see from these data that BRCA1 mutations may confer a higher risk of breast cancer, and a considerably higher risk of ovarian cancer, than BRCA2 mutations. In other words, BRCA1 mutations may be more penetrant than BRCA2 mutations.

BRCA gene mutations also become more penetrant with increasing age, meaning that cancers associated with these mutations are increasingly likely to manifest as we get older. This explains why there is a sharp rise in the incidence of breast and ovarian cancers in BRCA mutation carriers between the ages of 40 and 50 years. More specifically, the risk of ovarian cancer in women who carry a BRCA1 mutation rises significantly after age 40, and after age 45 for BRCA2, as can be seen in Table 2.

Research has shown that more recent generations are developing BRCA-related cancers at an earlier age than previous generations.[14] There may be many reasons for these differences, including, for example, diet, weight and exercise, the number of pregnancies a woman has had, her age at the time of pregnancy, as well as the role of other genes.

The Royal Marsden Hospital has also produced a table that details the risk of developing breast cancer according to age (see Table 3).

Table 3: Risk of developing breast cancer by age (women)

Current age	BRCA1		BRCA2	
	Approximate remaining lifetime risk to 80 years	Approximate 5 year risk	Approximate remaining lifetime risk to 80 years	Approximate 5 year risk
20–25	70%	5%	70%	1%
26–30	70%	5%	70%	2%
31–35	65%	5%	65%	5%
36–40	65%	10%	65%	5%
41–45	60%	10%	60%	10%
46–50	55%	15%	55%	10%
51–55	50%	15%	50%	10%
56–60	40%	10%	50%	10%
61–65	30%	10%	45%	15%
66–70	25%	10%	35%	15%

The Royal Marsden's *A Beginner's Guide to BRCA1 and BRCA2*[11]

Looking at these figures, we can see that the younger your age, the greater your approximate remaining lifetime risk is for developing breast cancer. For example, if you're 30 you have a large remaining risk for the rest of your lifetime, whereas if you're 65 you have a smaller remaining risk.

Between the ages of 56 and 70, the remaining lifetime risk of developing breast cancer is lower for BRCA1 mutation carriers than it is for BRCA2 mutation carriers. The reason for this is that BRCA1 mutations are more penetrant at younger ages than BRCA2 and, therefore, BRCA1-associated breast cancer tends to occur at a younger age than BRCA2. As a result, we see more cancers caused by inherited BRCA2 mutations in an ageing population.

Furthermore, the risk of developing cancer for BRCA2 carriers continues to increase throughout life, whereas in BRCA1 mutation carriers it appears to reduce initially and then level off with increasing age, as illustrated in Figure 6.

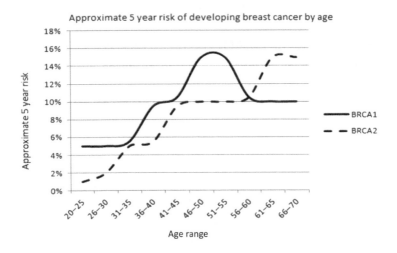

Figure 6: The risk of developing cancer for BRCA1 and BRCA2 mutation carriers, by age. (Data only taken from The Royal Marsden's *A Beginner's Guide to BRCA1 and BRCA2*[11])

We are still learning about the differences between the BRCA1 and BRCA2 genes; however, it has been shown that they are associated with different types of cancer. BRCA1 mutation carriers are more often diagnosed with aggressive forms of breast cancer that have not grown in response to hormones. On the other hand, BRCA2 carriers are more likely to develop breast cancer which has grown in response to oestrogen. Furthermore, BRCA2 mutation carriers are at greater risk than BRCA1 mutation carriers of developing other cancers including pancreatic, prostate cancer, and melanoma.

Cancer risk in men with BRCA mutations

In contrast to women, who have a greater lifetime risk of cancer with mutations of the BRCA1 gene, BRCA2 is the more important gene for men. Table 4 shows the cancer risks associated with BRCA1 and BRCA2 gene mutations in men.

Table 4: Cancer risks associated with BRCA1/2 Mutations in men

Gene	BRCA1	BRCA2
Male breast cancer, lifetime risk	0.1–1%	5–10%
Prostate cancer, lifetime risk	~10% – Similar to population risk	20–25%

The Royal Marsden's *A Beginner's Guide to BRCA1 and BRCA2*[11]

In general, male BRCA1 mutation carriers are at very low risk (0.1-1%) of breast cancer, whereas male BRCA2 mutation carriers have a 5-10% risk of developing breast cancer. Furthermore, male BRCA1 mutation carriers have a similar to population risk (approximately 10%) of developing prostate cancer, whereas BRCA2 mutation carriers have a much higher (20-25%) risk of developing this cancer.[11]

Further to the statistics above, it has been reported that the relative risk to male BRCA2 mutation carriers is high before age 65 years, and this is largely associated with breast, prostate and pancreatic cancers.[13] However, what is important to note here is that while a male BRCA2 mutation carrier has a high relative risk compared with that of a man in the general population, his absolute risk is still not that high. For example, a male BRCA2 mutation carrier has a 5-10% lifetime risk of breast cancer, but this is still considerably lower than a woman in the general population who has a 12.5% risk of breast cancer.

In contrast to women, relatively little is known about the risks for male BRCA mutation carriers. Additional research is necessary to gain a better understanding of these risks, particularly in relation to male BRCA2 mutation carriers.

Do different mutations have different risks?

In the last decade, several reports have been published supporting the hypothesis that different mutations in the BRCA1 or BRCA2 genes confer different cancer-related risks.

Evidence suggests that the Ashkenazi Jewish 'founder mutations' (BRCA1 185delAG, BRCA1 5382insC and BRCA2 6174delT – see page 17) are slightly less penetrant for both ovarian cancer and breast cancer than other BRCA gene mutations and, therefore, women with these particular mutations have considerably lower lifetime risks for breast and ovarian cancer compared with other BRCA mutation carriers.[15]

In particular, evidence suggests that carriers of the mutation BRCA2 6174delT have a lower risk of breast cancer compared with other BRCA2 gene mutations.[16] Ashkenazi Jewish families with the 6174delT founder mutation are more likely to have a family member with ovarian cancer compared with other BRCA2 gene mutations.[17] In contrast, a reduced incidence of ovarian cancer has been found in families of French-Canadian ancestry, compared with other ancestries.[17] The BRCA2 6503delTT mutation often seen in Ireland and Scotland, but which is also seen throughout Europe and the USA, appears to confer a high risk of male breast cancer.[17] Evidence suggests that families of Polish ancestry have a reduced risk of pancreatic cancer compared with families of other ethnic origins.[17] In conclusion, both the position of the mutation and the ethnic background of the family appear to contribute to the type of cancer observed in families with BRCA mutations.[17]

Some evidence suggests the possibility that mutations in specific regions of the BRCA1 and BRCA2 genes may confer higher risks of breast or ovarian cancer than other regions. These regions have been termed the 'ovarian cancer cluster region' (OCCR) and the 'breast cancer cluster region' (BCCR). However, there has been some debate within the scientific community as to whether these regions actually exist, so caution is advised when considering these regions whilst deciding on risk-reducing strategies.

The ovarian cancer cluster region (OCCR)

The ovarian cancer cluster region refers to a region of the BRCA1 and BRCA2 genes in which mutations have been observed to confer an increased risk of ovarian cancer and a decreased risk of breast cancer. However, it is important to note that patients who carry mutations within the OCCR have developed breast cancer and, likewise, patients whose mutations sit outside of the OCCR have developed ovarian cancer.

A large study by Rebbeck et al, published in 2015, aimed to identify mutation-specific cancer risks for carriers of BRCA1/2 mutations. According to the findings of this study, BRCA1 is thought to contain a single OCCR found in the central portion of the gene within exon 11 between nucleotides c.1380 and c.4062.[18] Mutations in this part of the gene are associated with increased ovarian cancer risk, but decreased breast cancer risk.

Furthermore, for BRCA1, mutations in exon 11 were associated with an earlier age at diagnosis for either cancer.

BRCA1 mutation carriers are usually considered to have a higher risk of ovarian cancer than BRCA2 mutation carriers, but mutations in the ovarian cancer cluster region of BRCA2 may actually confer nearly as high a risk as BRCA1. The BRCA2 gene contains three OCCRs: the first spanned c.3249 to c.5681, which was adjacent to mutation c.5946delT (6174delT), and the second OCCR spanned c.6645 to c.7471. Mutations which lie within these regions, including 6174delT, are associated with a higher ovarian cancer risk and a lower breast cancer risk compared with other BRCA2 gene mutations.[18, 16] However, an earlier study, published in 2001, reported that the optimal definition of the BRCA2 OCCR was bounded by slightly different nucleotides: 3059-4075 and 6503-6629. OCCR mutations were associated both with a highly significantly decreased risk of breast cancer and with a significantly increased risk of ovarian cancer.[19]

Breast cancer cluster region (BCCR)

Similarly, the breast cancer cluster region (BCCR) is a region of the BRCA1 and BRCA2 genes in which mutations have been observed to confer an increased risk of breast cancer and a decreased risk of ovarian cancer. However, as with the OCCR, patients who carry mutations within the BCCR have also developed ovarian cancer and, similarly, patients whose mutations sit outside of this BCCR have developed breast cancer. Caution is, once again, advised when considering these regions whilst deciding on risk-reducing strategies.

According to the findings of the study by Rebbeck et al, the BRCA1 and BRCA2 gene both harbour three breast cancer cluster regions. For BRCA1, these are located at c.179 to c.505, c.4328 to c.4945 and c.5261 to c.5563. The common founder Jewish mutation c.5266dupC, better known as BRCA1 5382insC, lies within the breast cancer cluster region of the BRCA1 gene.

In BRCA2, multiple BCCRs spanning c.1 to c.596, c.772 to c.1806 and c.7394 to c.8904 have been observed.[18] For BRCA2, researchers note a later age at breast cancer diagnosis in women whose mutations were in the OCCR regions, and earlier onset for mutations in the BCCR regions.[18]

In summary, Dr Rebbeck explained: 'Mutations in extreme regions [the ends] of the BRCA1 gene are more likely to increase susceptibility to breast cancer and mutations in the central portion of the gene, around exon 11, are more likely to increase susceptibility to ovarian cancer.'[3] If it were possible to determine precise levels of risk for each mutation found within the BRCA1 and BRCA2 gene, it would have important implications for screening, genetic counselling and risk-reducing treatment. Furthermore, if it were possible to make an accurate prediction of the most likely age that cancer would occur for mutations, then this 'might have important implications for the timing of prevention strategies. If diagnosis would likely be early, around age 30, a woman might be more likely to have oophorectomy than a woman who would be predicted to be diagnosed at age 50 and can maintain fertility as long as possible,' said Dr Rebbeck.[3]

Misconceptions about the BRCA gene

Perhaps the most common misconception is that not everyone carries a BRCA1 and BRCA2 gene. This is false – we all have the gene. If a patient is BRCA-positive this doesn't mean they carry the BRCA gene, it means they carry a harmful mutation that stops the gene from functioning properly. If a patient is BRCA-negative, then they do not carry a harmful mutation in their BRCA gene and their gene will function properly as a tumour suppressor, thereby helping to prevent cancer developing.

- **If I test positive for a BRCA gene mutation, does that mean I will get cancer?** No, it does not. Carrying a

BRCA gene mutation means that there is an increased risk of developing cancers associated with these mutations, but it does not mean that you definitely will develop cancer. Not all women who inherit a BRCA mutation will develop breast or ovarian cancer. Likewise, not all men who inherit a BRCA mutation will develop breast or prostate cancer. The reason for this variation in risk is thought to be dependent on 'lifestyle factors' such as smoking and dietary influences, as well as the inheritance of other cancer susceptibility genes, and a certain element of chance.

- **Can a BRCA gene mutation skip a generation?** The answer to this question is 'No'. BRCA gene mutations do not skip generations. However, it sometimes looks like the cancer has skipped a generation when considering family history. The reason for this is that, even though having a BRCA gene mutation increases the chance of developing cancer, some people with the mutation never get the disease. This is especially true when the gene mutation is passed through a male, who will have a lower risk of cancer than a woman who carries the gene mutation. For example, it's possible to have a family history in which a woman and her father's mother both develop breast cancer due to a BRCA gene mutation, but the woman's father does not develop cancer. It may appear as if it has skipped the father; however, in reality he carries the mutation but, for reasons unknown, in his case it doesn't lead to cancer. A small family size or early death from other causes may also obscure predisposition to cancer within a family.

- **Can we switch off the BRCA gene to prevent cancer?** Some claim that the risk of cancer in BRCA gene mutation carriers can be controlled by 'turning the

BRCA gene on and off'. This is wrong and misleading. Carriers of a BRCA gene mutation are at risk of cancer because their gene cannot work properly as a tumour suppressor. The mutated gene either produces no tumour suppressor protein at all, or it produces one which isn't able to suppress the formation of a tumour. Simply turning this gene on or off, even if it were possible, would have no effect on this cancer risk because, when a mutation is present, the gene no longer works as it should and it loses its ability to suppress cancer.

- **If I test negative for a BRCA gene mutation, does that mean I will not get cancer?** The answer to this question is 'No'. There are many factors that contribute to a person developing cancer. In fact, only 3-5% of women with breast cancer carry a BRCA gene mutation.[8] The majority of breast cancer cases are 'sporadic', meaning there is no definitive gene mutation. Cancer is a 'multifactorial' disease, which means that it is caused by a combination of many factors, including both genetic and environmental. Even if you do not carry a BRCA gene mutation, you may still be at increased risk of developing cancer depending upon the cause of the cancer in your family.

Evolutionary advantage of BRCA mutations

In the natural course of evolution, harmful genes should have been eliminated from the human population over time. Any gene that doesn't help people survive, reproduce and rear their children to an age where they too can reproduce and pass on their genes will eventually be removed from the population. However, BRCA mutations have persisted across generations and, from the standpoint of evolution, for a harmful mutation such as BRCA1/2 to be maintained in the population, there is likely to be some potential evolutionary advantage to having it. However, it is important to bear in mind that the fundamental reason why BRCA gene mutations have persisted across generations is because carriers tend to survive long enough to be able to pass on their genes to successive generations.

One proposed, although highly controversial, theory is that these BRCA mutations increase intelligence. The Ashkenazi intelligence hypothesis, proposed by Gregory Cochran et al, suggests that a mutation in the BRCA1 gene leads to greater neural growth within the human brain which, in turn, leads to increased intelligence.[20] However, other scientists have given Cochran's theory a mixed reception, ranging from outright dismissal to acknowledgement that the hypothesis might be true and merits further research.[21]

Besides the possibility of superior intelligence, mutated BRCA genes may also offer an important evolutionary advantage of increased lactation.[22] The role of the normal copy of the gene is to control cell proliferation in the breasts, ovaries and prostate, but a mutation which knocks that out of control could allow for increased lactation. This increased lactation would have been a benefit to societies living on meagre diets providing barely enough for survival. However, it is unlikely to be beneficial to young women in the modern era.

Scientists have also explored the idea that increased fertility might be a potential advantage in BRCA mutations.[23] Using information collected from the Utah Population Database (UPDB), a team of researchers looked at patterns of both childbearing and early death in two groups of women with BRCA1/2 mutations representing two eras. They also looked at control groups who did not carry the mutation. One group consisted of women born before 1930, who would have completed their childbearing years before birth control was readily available and reliable. The other group included women from later generations who had access to effective birth control. The researchers found that having a BRCA1/2 mutation enhances fertility: women with the mutation who lived during a time when they did not have access to birth control had significantly more children than women without the mutation. For BRCA1/2 carriers who lived when access to effective birth control was available, the fertility difference persisted but it was not as large. At the same time, the study showed that, in their post-reproductive years, more mutation carriers died at earlier ages than women without BRCA mutations.[23] This research shows that mutations are both harmful and beneficial which, in turn, offers a possible explanation as to why these BRCA mutations continue to be prevalent in the population. Interestingly, however, some research suggests that BRCA1 gene mutations may actually decrease fertility, although this effect was not seen in BRCA2 mutation carriers.[24, 25]

Section III

Cancer and its relationship with BRCA gene mutations

This section aims to improve your understanding of what cancer is, followed by a closer look at those cancers which are strongly associated with BRCA gene mutations, including breast, ovarian and prostate cancer. This section also covers uterine cancer and whether or not BRCA gene mutation carriers may be at increased risk of developing this disease. Lastly, this section looks at the other cancers which BRCA mutation carriers may be at a slightly increased risk of developing, such as pancreatic cancer and melanoma.

5.

Cancer

According to Cancer Research UK, one in two people born after 1960 in the UK will be diagnosed with some form of cancer during their lifetime.[1] More than 352,000 people are diagnosed with cancer in the UK each year – a 12% increase in the rate since the mid-90s.[2] This rise is mainly due to the ageing and growing population and, while the chances of getting cancer have increased, the chances of surviving it have also improved. In addition to this, this rise is also likely to result from the fact that with the advent of modern antibiotics, fewer people are dying from infectious diseases and, therefore, people are living longer and, hence, getting cancer.

What is cancer?

The term 'cancer' encompasses a large collection of illnesses that have one essential trait in common: a loss of cell cycle control. That is, a cell divides again and again when it should not and each time it divides mutations are likely to occur. Mutations are occurring all the time within our cells and can be harmless; however, continued mutations within a cell can give rise to cancer.

Before we take a look at cancer, let's distinguish between benign and malignant tumours. Tumours are groups of abnormal cells that form lumps or growths. Tumours which are benign are not cancerous, but they still suggest that there has been a loss of cell cycle control as, normally, cell division should be switched off at the appropriate point, preventing the development of a tumour. Benign tumours are not typically life-threatening in themselves, and they do not have the ability to spread around the body.

Cancer begins with a single abnormal cell that continues to divide to produce others like itself. These cells may grow into a mass called a malignant tumour. They tend to grow quite a lot faster than benign tumours and these cells can break away from the primary site and spread to other parts of the body. These cells can attach to other tissues and organs to form secondary cancers or metastases (pronounced met-as-tah-seez) in other sites within the body. Cancer cells may arise in everyone, probably because cell division occurs so frequently that an occasional cell escapes the mechanisms that normally control the process. The immune system destroys most cancer cells, but a few may survive and lead to the formation of a malignant tumour.

How cancers get bigger

When cancer first develops, the cancer cells are contained within the body tissue in which they have developed – for example within the breast ducts. There is a non-invasive form of breast cancer which is commonly referred to as 'carcinoma in situ' and, if it has developed within the breast ducts, it is diagnosed as Ductal Carcinoma in Situ, or DCIS for short. It is this type of cancer which tends to develop within the breasts of BRCA muta-tion carriers. We will take a more detailed look at this later on in the 'Breast Cancer' section of this book (page 60).

Some body tissues have a layer, called the 'basement membrane', which keeps the cells of that tissue inside it. One of the functions of this membrane is to act as a barrier to prevent malignant cells from reaching and invading deeper tissues. Once the cancer cells have broken through this membrane it is called an invasive cancer.

Superficial carcinoma in situ, such as DCIS, has the potential to become invasive cancer, although this does not always occur. Invasive breast cancer is very serious as it is potentially life-threatening.

Blood supply and cancer

As the tumour grows, the centre of it gets further away from the blood vessels which are supplying it with oxygen and other nutrients which are vital for its survival. It is harder for the oxygen to reach the centre of the tumour, as shown in Figure 7.

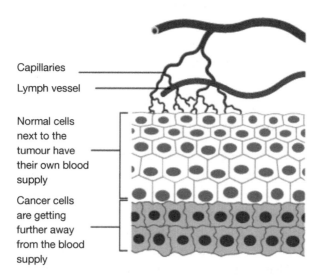

Capillaries

Lymph vessel

Normal cells next to the tumour have their own blood supply

Cancer cells are getting further away from the blood supply

Figure 7: How cancer grows[3]

Cells cannot survive without this oxygen and nutrients and will endeavour to send out signals, known as 'angiogenic factors'. These angiogenic factors encourage new blood vessels to grow into the tumour. This process is called 'angiogenesis'. Without a blood supply, the tumour would grow no larger than a pin head in size. Once a cancer can stimulate blood vessel growth, it will receive enough oxygen and other nutrients to enable it to grow bigger, and to do so much more quickly.

Scientists have found very large amounts of angiogenic factors at the outer edges of a cancer. For example, breast and ovarian cancers are associated with high concentrations of vascular endothelial growth factor (VEGF), which is a protein that stimulates the growth of new blood vessels.

How cancer spreads

Spreading into surrounding tissues

As a tumour gets bigger, it takes up more room in the body. The cancer can then cause pressure on surrounding organs and it can also grow directly into body structures nearby. This is called 'local invasion'.

A cancer may just grow out in a random direction from the place where it started. However, tumours can spread into some tissues more easily than others. For example, large blood vessels which have very strong walls and dense tissues such as cartilage are hard for tumours to grow into. As a result, tumours tend to grow along the path of least resistance – such as growing between sheets of muscle tissue rather than straight through a muscle.

As the tumour grows and takes up more space, it begins to press on the normal body tissue nearby. The tumour growth will force itself through the normal tissue, as in Figure 8.

As the cancer grows, it may squeeze and block small blood vessels in the area. Because of the resulting low blood and oxygen levels, some of the normal tissue will begin to die off, making it easier for the cancer to continue to push its way through. This dead tissue must be cleared away so that the body can replace it with new, healthy tissue. Our white blood cells produce chemicals called enzymes which break down the tissue.

These same enzymes can also be used to attack invading bacteria and viruses. This is all part of the natural healing process which occurs in our bodies.

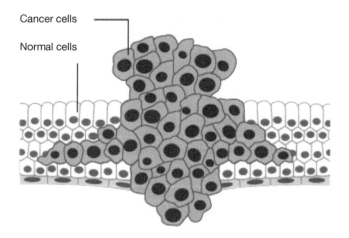

Figure 8: Cancer grows as cells multiply over and over[4]

As part of the body's immune response to cancer, some cancers contain a lot of normal white blood cells, which produce these enzymes. Many cancers contain larger amounts of these enzymes than normal tissues and these enzymes are, in fact, likely to make it easier for the cancer to grow through the healthy tissue. In addition to this, cancerous cells produce a substance which stimulates these cells to move about. Cancer cells don't stick together as well as normal cells do and can, therefore, easily break away and spread to other areas of the body.

Spreading to other areas of the body

Cancer cells can be carried in the bloodstream or lymphatic system to other parts of the body, where they can then grow into new tumours. Figure 9 shows a tumour appearing in cells lining a body structure. The tumour grows through the basement membrane which normally holds the cells in place. Some cells can then move into small lymph vessels or blood vessels called capillaries in the area.

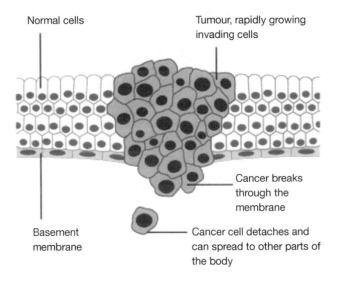

Normal cells

Tumour, rapidly growing invading cells

Cancer breaks through the membrane

Basement membrane

Cancer cell detaches and can spread to other parts of the body

Figure 9: How cancer can spread[5]

Spreading through the blood circulation

If the cancer cells go into small blood vessels they can then get into the bloodstream; they are called circulating tumour cells. The circulating blood sweeps the cancer cells along until they get stuck somewhere. Usually they get stuck in a very small blood vessel, such as a capillary (see Figure 10).

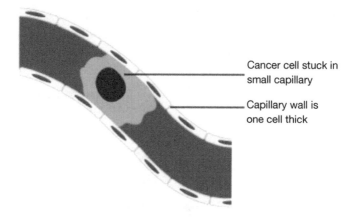

Figure 10: Spread through the blood circulation[5]

The cell must then move through the wall of the capillary, which is very thin (only one cell thick), and into the tissue of the organ close by (see Figure 11). If the conditions are right and the cell has nutrients, such as oxygen and sugar, it can multiply to form a new tumour.

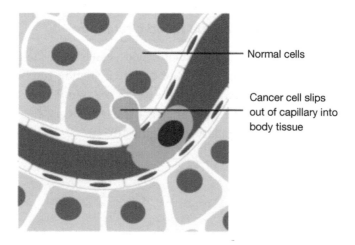

Figure 11: Spreading to other tissues[5]

This is quite a complicated journey and most cancer cells don't survive it, either because they are destroyed by the white blood cells in our immune system, or because they are battered around by the fast-flowing blood. Probably, out of many thousands of cancer cells that reach the blood circulation, only a few will survive to form a secondary cancer.

Spread through the lymphatic system

The lymphatic system consists of thin tubes, called lymph vessels, and lymph nodes that run throughout the body. The lymph vessels contain a colourless fluid (lymph) which holds a high number of white blood cells.

If cancer cells go into the small lymph vessels close to the primary tumour, they can be carried through these vessels and into nearby lymph nodes, where they may 'get stuck'. In the lymph nodes (glands) they may be destroyed, but some may survive and grow to form tumours in one or more lymph nodes. Doctors call this 'lymph node spread'. If the surrounding lymph nodes are found to contain any cancer cells this shows that cancer cells have broken away from the original cancer site and travelled as far as the nodes, but it is very difficult to know whether these cells have spread beyond these nodes into other areas of the body.

Determining whether a cancer has spread elsewhere in the body is important for doctors in deciding on the best course of treatment for a cancer. Doctors may perform tests to determine the stage of the cancer. If it is likely that the cancer has spread (it is at an advanced stage), doctors may offer extra treatment, such as chemotherapy or radiotherapy, to decrease the probability of recurrence.

6.
Breast cancer

The breasts are made up of fat, connective tissue and thousands of tiny glands called 'lobules', which produce milk (see Figure 12). While the breasts have a role in sexual arousal, their main function is to produce milk ready to feed a newborn baby. Hormonal changes in late pregnancy stimulate the production of milk in the lobules. This breast milk is then carried through tiny tubes called 'ducts' to the nipple, ready for breastfeeding.

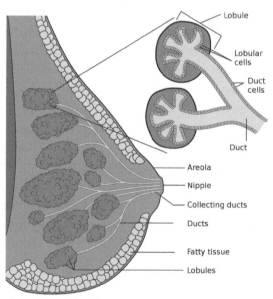

Figure 12: The normal breast

Breast cancer is the most common type of cancer in the UK, except for skin cancer.[6] It is also the most frequently diagnosed cancer and the leading cause of cancer death among females worldwide.[7] Every year nearly 62,000 women and 390 men are diagnosed with breast cancer in the UK, the equivalent of one person every 10 minutes. Around 11,400 people die from breast cancer in the UK every year.[8] Breast cancer is also the most common cancer among American women (except for skin cancers). In the US, it is estimated that about 252,710 cases of invasive breast cancer will be diagnosed in women in 2017. It is also estimated in the US that in the same year, about 40,610 women will die from the disease.[9]

The good news is that breast cancer survival rates are improving in the western world, and they have been for the last 30 years. This is largely due to screening, earlier diagnosis and improved treatments.[9,10] The earlier breast cancer is caught, the better chance a person has of surviving five years after being diagnosed. According to Cancer Research UK, 96% of women survive breast cancer for at least one year, 87% of women are expected to survive the disease for five years or more and 78% of women are predicted to survive their disease for ten years or more.[11]

As mentioned in Chapter 4, page 37 in the UK, 12.5% of women (one in eight) in the general population will develop breast cancer sometime during their lifetime. However, breast cancer does occur more often than usual in some families because of their genetic make-up. By contrast, 60-90% of women who inherit a harmful BRCA1 mutation and 45-85% of women who inherit a harmful BRCA2 mutation will develop breast cancer during their lifetime.[12]

Again as mentioned in Chapter 4, only 3-5% of all breast cancer cases are due to inherited BRCA gene mutations.[13] The vast majority are the result of biological and environmental factors to which women are exposed. Simply being a woman is the main risk factor for developing breast cancer, along with getting older and having a significant family history.

In the general population, the majority of women diagnosed with breast cancer are over 50. However, women with BRCA gene mutations are more likely to develop breast cancer at a younger age. In addition, breast cancer in these women more often affects both breasts than cancers not linked to these mutations. BRCA mutation carriers who have had breast cancer also have a higher risk of developing another new breast cancer, compared with women in the general population.[12] Furthermore, BRCA1-related breast cancer tends to be more aggressive than normal breast cancer; however, evidence suggests little or no difference in survival rates between sporadic and BRCA1/2-associated breast cancer.[14, 15]

According to the World Health Organization, the global increase in breast cancer incidence is due to many factors, including reproductive history, genetics, radiation (especially at times of breast development) and the Western lifestyle with a high calorie diet, obesity and lack of physical activity.[16] More specifically, increased risk is linked to the following, according to Cancer Research UK[17] and other sources:

- starting periods (menarche) before the age of 12;
- not having children or having a first pregnancy at the age of 30 or older;
- a lack of breastfeeding;
- menopause later than the average age of 51 years;
- long-term use of oral contraceptives or hormonal replacement therapy (HRT);
- being overweight;
- lack of exercise;
- drinking alcohol;
- getting older;
- family history of breast cancer;
- BRCA1 or BRCA2 gene mutations.

In the general population, early menarche and late menopause are important risk factors for breast cancer. For a woman in the general population, the earlier her age at first menarche and the later her age at menopause, the higher her risk is of developing breast cancer because she will be exposed to oestrogen, known to fuel the growth and initiate the development of some breast cancers, for a longer period of time. These effects are broadly similar for BRCA mutation carriers.

There are a number of reproductive factors which may decrease the risk of breast cancer in the general population. These include starting a family at a younger age, having a greater than average number of children and breastfeeding for more than one year. However, with regard to BRCA mutation carriers, these factors may not offer the same protection. A study published in 2005 reported that the risk of breast cancer in BRCA1 mutation carriers did not decrease with pregnancy until after four births, after which there was only a modest protective effect. In contrast, for BRCA2 mutation carriers, there was a statistically significant increase in breast cancer risk with each additional pregnancy.[18]

In relation to age of first giving birth, evidence suggests that having a child at a young age does not protect against breast cancer for BRCA1/2 mutation carriers.[19, 20] Furthermore, a meta-analysis of 10 studies published in 2014 found that late age at first birth protects against breast cancer in BRCA1, but not BRCA2, mutation carriers.[21]

With regard to breastfeeding, a large international study of women with breast cancer in the general population found that the risk of breast cancer was reduced by 4.3% for women who had breastfed for 12 months or more and by 27% for women who had breastfed for 55 months or more. In other words, the longer women breastfeed the more they are protected against breast cancer.[22] Similarly, evidence suggests that for BRCA1 mutation carriers, breastfeeding for at least one year is associated with a significant reduction in breast cancer risk; breastfeeding for two or more years leads to a greater reduction in risk. However, among BRCA2 mutation carriers, there was no significant association between breastfeeding and breast cancer risk. In conclusion, breastfeeding protects against BRCA1- but not BRCA2-associated breast cancer.[23]

In the general population, oral contraceptives have been associated with a small increased breast cancer risk, which tends to level off a few years after use has ceased. Reassuringly, a meta-analysis of 18 studies published in 2010 found no evidence of a significant association between recent oral contraceptives and breast cancer risk in BRCA1/2 carriers. However, oral contraceptive formulations used before 1975 (when, on average, the oestrogen content was higher than that in oral contraceptives produced after 1975) were associated with a significant increased risk of breast cancer.[24]

With regard to hormone replacement therapy (HRT), evidence suggests that even relatively short-term combined HRT, containing both oestrogen and progesterone, after a natural menopause increases the risk of breast cancer compared with women who do not take HRT.[25] The longer the duration of therapy, the higher the risk conferred. However, once women stop taking HRT their risk goes back to normal within five years.[12] It is unclear if this same effect occurs in BRCA mutation carriers. However, evidence suggests that women who take HRT in the short term to manage menopausal symptoms after risk-reducing removal of their ovaries still benefit from a reduction in breast cancer risk despite taking HRT.[26]

Symptoms of breast cancer

The symptoms which may occur in breast cancer are:
- a lump or thickening in an area of the breast;
- a change in the size, shape or feel of a breast;
- a dimpling of the skin;

- a change in the shape of the nipple, particularly if it turns in, sinks into the breast, or has an irregular shape;
- a bloodstained discharge from the nipple;
- a rash on a nipple or surrounding area;
- a swelling or lump in the armpit.

These signs may also occur in benign conditions but, if there are any changes from what is normal for you, book an appointment with your family doctor. Seeing a doctor early also means that if it does turn out to be cancer, you are giving yourself the best chance of successful treatment.

Types of breast cancer

Breast cancers arise from the epithelial cells which line the ducts and lobules (see Figure 12). There are many different types of breast cancer which can develop in different parts of the breast. Breast cancer is often divided into non-invasive and invasive types.

Non-invasive breast cancer

Non-invasive breast cancer is also known as cancer or carcinoma in situ. This cancer is found in the ducts of the breast and hasn't developed the ability to spread outside the breast. This form of cancer rarely shows as a lump in the breast and is usually detected by an MRI or a mammogram. The most common type of non-invasive cancer is 'ductal carcinoma in situ' (DCIS). Doctors may describe DCIS as a very early form of breast cancer, often referred to as 'stage 0 breast cancer'. It may also be referred to as pre-invasive, non-invasive, ductal intraepithelial neoplasia (DIN) or intra-ductal cancer.

A diagnosis of DCIS means that cells inside some of the breast ducts have turned into cancer cells. There is very little chance that any of these cancerous cells would have spread to the lymph nodes or other areas of the body. DCIS isn't considered to be life-threatening but, if it is not treated, in some women it may start to spread into the surrounding breast tissue and progress into invasive breast cancer. Currently, there is no good way to know for certain which cases will go on to become invasive cancers and which ones won't.

According to Cancer Research UK, around 5100 people are diagnosed with DCIS in the UK each year, of which about 15 are men.[27] According to the American Cancer Society, about 60,000 American women are diagnosed with DCIS each year, accounting for about one out of every five new breast cancer cases.[28] The main reason why this number is so large, and has been increasing over time, is because people are living much longer and, as we grow older, our risk of breast cancer increases. In addition, more people are having mammograms and, therefore, more cancers are being spotted early. Furthermore, with the recent introduction of digital mammography, more cases of DCIS are being detected and diagnosed.

Invasive breast cancer

Invasive breast cancer is cancer that spreads outside the basement membrane of the lobule, or duct, into the breast tissue. In 2014, more than 55,000 women in the UK were diagnosed with invasive breast cancer.[29] According to the American Cancer Society, more than 180,000 women in the United States are diagnosed with invasive breast cancer each year.[30] Invasive cancer can spread to other parts of the body, usually through the lymph nodes or bloodstream. When breast cancer cells are found in other parts of the body, the cancer is called 'metastatic breast cancer'.

The two most common types of invasive breast cancer are 'invasive ductal carcinoma' (IDC) and 'invasive lobular carcinoma' (ILC).

IDC, which develops in the cells that line the breast ducts, accounts for about 80% of all breast cancer cases.[31] A type of IDC typically seen in BRCA1 mutation carriers is known as 'basal' or 'basal-like' breast cancer. This form of IDC arises in the basal cells lining the breast ducts and accounts for up to 15% of all breast cancers.[32]

ILC develops in the cells that line the milk-producing lobules and accounts for about 10% of invasive breast cancers.[31]

Inflammatory breast cancer (IBC) is another, but less common, type of invasive breast cancer which may also arise in BRCA mutation carriers.[33] Inflammatory breast cancer is rare, but it is the most aggressive form of breast cancer, typically characterised by a swollen red breast often with an inverted nipple and no lump. The skin over the breast is warm and thickened, with a 'peau d'orange' – skin of an orange – appearance.

Classifying breast cancer based on hormone receptors and HER2 status

Doctors often divide invasive breast cancers into groups based on the presence of hormone and protein receptors. Hormones or other proteins can attach to these receptors and stimulate the cancer to grow, so classifying cancers in this way helps doctors to understand how a tumour may act and what kind of treatments may work best.

The hormones oestrogen and progesterone attach to oestrogen and progesterone receptors (ER and PR) respectively, while the protein HER2 (human epidermal growth factor receptor 2) attaches to HER2 receptors. Some breast cancers have one or more of these receptors, while breast cancers which are triple negative don't have any of them (so-called hormone-receptor negative tumours).

Hormone receptors

About 80% of breast cancers are ER positive, of which about 65%

are also progesterone-receptor positive.[34] If a breast cancer has a significant number of receptors for either oestrogen or progesterone, it is considered hormone-receptor positive. Tumours that are ER/PR-positive are much more likely to respond to hormone therapy with drugs, such as tamoxifen, which block the effects of oestrogen, than tumours that are ER/PR-negative.

Breast cancer in BRCA2 carriers is more likely to be oestrogen-receptor-positive, meaning that they are more likely to develop breast cancer that is fuelled by oestrogen. If the breast cancer cells have neither oestrogen nor progesterone receptors, they are said to be hormone receptor-negative. These cancers tend to grow more quickly than hormone receptor-positive cancers and, if they return, it is more often in the first few years.

Protein receptors

In about 20% of breast cancers, the cells make too much HER2. These cancers tend to be aggressive and fast-growing.[34] For women with HER2-positive breast cancers, the drug trastuzumab (Herceptin) has been shown to dramatically reduce the risk of the cancer coming back. This drug is given with chemotherapy for early-stage breast cancer or for metastatic breast cancer (breast cancer which has spread to other areas of the body). Trastuzumab has far fewer immediate side-effects than chemotherapy – for example, there is usually no nausea or hair loss – but side-effects may include headaches, diarrhoea and, infrequently, heart damage.

Triple positive / Triple negative

Cancers that are ER-positive, PR-positive, and have too much HER2 are called triple-positive breast cancer. These cancers are treated with hormone drugs as well as drugs that target HER2.

If the cancer does not have receptors for either HER2 or for oestrogen and progesterone, it is called triple-negative breast cancer. Triple negative accounts for up to 15% of women with breast cancer and is more common in younger, premenopausal women.[32]

Most breast cancers associated with the BRCA1 gene are triple negative (basal-like breast cancer), but triple negative breast cancers may also be seen in BRCA2 mutation carriers. Currently in the UK, any woman under the age of 50 who is diagnosed with grade three triple-negative breast cancer is routinely tested for a BRCA gene mutation. Triple-negative breast cancer tumours are among the most aggressive – they grow fast and spread quickly, making them more likely than other types of cancer to be life-threatening. Hormone therapies, such as tamoxifen, and anti-HER2 therapies, such as trastuzumab (Herceptin), are not effective against these cancers.

However, triple-negative breast cancer patients with BRCA mutations appear to have better survival rates than patients who have triple-negative breast cancer without a BRCA gene mutation.[35]

7.
Male breast cancer

Many people don't know that men can get breast cancer because they don't think of men as having breasts. In fact, both men and women have breast tissue, although men have much smaller amounts than women. Men's breast tissue has ducts, but only a few, if any, lobules (see Figure 13).

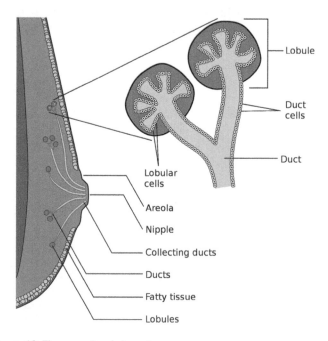

Figure 13: The normal male breast

Like all cells in the body, a man's breast ducts can undergo cancerous changes. However, breast cancer is less common in men because their ducts are less developed than those of women, and they normally have lower levels of the female hormones that can trigger the onset of breast cancer.

Male breast cancer is a very rare and poorly understood disease. There are about 390 men diagnosed with breast cancer each year in the UK, compared with around 62,000 cases of breast cancer in women.[36] Most men who get breast cancer are over 60, although younger men can be affected.[36] In the US, about 2470 new cases of invasive breast cancer are expected to be diagnosed in men in 2017 and about 460 men will die from the disease.[37]

Men in the UK have about a one in 1000 or 0.1% chance of developing breast cancer in their lifetime. According to Cancer Research UK, male breast cancer incidence has remained stable in Great Britain since the late 1970s.[29] By contrast, up to 1% of men who inherit a harmful BRCA1 mutation and between 5 and 10% of men who inherit a harmful BRCA2 mutation will develop breast cancer during their lifetime.[12]

Approximately half of the men who develop breast cancer have a mutation in a BRCA gene or in one of the other genes associated with hereditary breast–ovarian cancer syndromes. BRCA2 mutation is the strongest risk factor for male breast cancer and men with these mutations have a dramatically elevated risk of developing the disease. While BRCA1 carriers are at lower risk than BRCA2 carriers, they are at increased risk compared with the general population. A study published in 2007 estimated that the cumulative risk of breast cancer at age 70 was 1.2% for male BRCA1 mutation carriers and 6.8% for male BRCA2 mutation carriers.[38]

Although the exact causes of breast cancer in men are not fully understood, certain factors may increase the risk. The most important risk factor is age. In fact, very few men, with or without a predisposing mutation, develop breast cancer before the age of 50 and most cases are diagnosed in men between the ages of 60 and 70.[39] Male breast cancers associated with BRCA2 mutations are, however, typically diagnosed at a younger age.

Other risk factors include exposure to high oestrogen levels and exposure to radiation. Men produce small amounts of oestrogen in their testes, adrenal glands and liver. However, men who are very overweight are likely to be exposed to much higher levels of oestrogen because it is also partly made in the fat (adipose) tissues of the body. It is well known that high oestrogen levels are linked to breast cancer.

Men who have been exposed to radiation repeatedly, especially from a young age and over a long period of time, are more likely to develop breast cancer.

As with women, most male breast cancer cells have hormone receptors. About 90% are oestrogen receptor (ER) positive and about 81% are progesterone receptor (PR) positive.[40]

Symptoms of breast cancer in men

The most common symptom for men with breast cancer is normally a painless lump in the breast area. Other symptoms can include:

- oozing from the nipple (a discharge) that may be bloodstained;
- swelling of the breast;
- a sore (ulcer) in the skin of the breast;
- a nipple that is pulled into the breast (called nipple retraction);
- lumps under the arm.

As in women, these signs may occur in benign conditions, but if there are any changes from what is normal for you, it's important to see your family doctor. Seeking medical help early on also means that, if it does turn out to be cancer, there will be a higher probability of successful treatment.

Types of breast cancer

The most common type of breast cancer in men is invasive ductal carcinoma (IDC). However, as is true for women, men can be diagnosed with non-invasive ductal carcinoma in situ (DCIS).

Non-invasive breast cancer

Non-invasive breast cancer is also known as cancer or carcinoma in situ. This cancer is found in the ducts of the breast and hasn't developed the ability to spread outside the breast.

As stated previously, approximately 15 cases of DCIS occur each year in men in the UK.[27] DCIS accounts for about one in 10 cases of breast cancer in men and it is almost always curable with surgery.[41]

Invasive breast cancer

Invasive breast cancer is cancer that spreads outside the membrane of the lobule or duct into the breast tissue. The cancer can then spread into the lymph nodes in the armpit or beyond. The two most common types of invasive breast cancer are invasive ductal carcinoma (IDC) and invasive lobular carcinoma (ILC). At least eight out of 10 male breast cancers are IDCs (alone or mixed with other types of invasive or in situ breast cancer).[41] Because the male breast is much smaller than the female breast, all male breast cancers start relatively close to the nipple, so they are more likely to spread to the nipple. ILC is very rare in men, accounting for only about 2% of male breast cancers.[41] This is because men do not usually have much lobular tissue.

Breast cancer in men can be treated as successfully as breast cancer in women, but men often ignore the signs and symptoms.

Overall, survival rates for male breast cancer are lower than for female breast cancers due to the older age and more advanced disease at the time of diagnosis. However, because the incidence of male breast cancer is so low, there are not enough data to provide accurate survival rate statistics.[10]

Currently in the UK, men who carry BRCA mutations are not offered breast screening, or risk-reducing surgery to remove their breast tissue, but are instead advised to examine their breasts regularly and to seek advice from their family doctor if they are at all concerned.

8.
Ovarian cancer

The ovaries are a pair of small organs in the female reproductive system that contain and release an egg once a month. This process is known as ovulation. Figure 14 is a diagram of the female reproductive system showing the position of the ovaries.

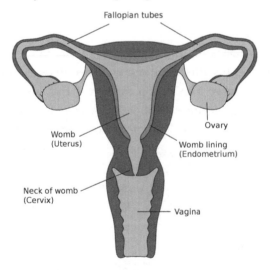

Figure 14: The female reproductive system

Ovarian cancer is the leading cause of death from gynaecological cancers in the UK. It kills around 4000 women each year in the UK and is usually diagnosed at an advanced stage, with just 40% of patients surviving five years after diagnosis.[42] In the US, ovarian cancer is also the most lethal gynaecological cancer and is responsible for as many as 13,000 deaths per year.[43]

Ovarian cancer is most often diagnosed in women who are between 40 and 60 years of age, although it can affect women of any age. Most women who develop ovarian cancer have few symptoms until the cancer has spread, at which point the cancer is more difficult to treat. However, treatment is often successful in women who are diagnosed during the earliest stages of the disease.

In the UK, around 7100 women are diagnosed with ovarian cancer each year.[44] In the general population, approximately 2% of women will get ovarian cancer in their lifetime.[45] However, as many as 40-60% of women who inherit a harmful BRCA1 mutation and 10-30% of women who inherit a harmful BRCA2 mutation will develop ovarian cancer during their lifetime.[12] BRCA1 and BRCA2 mutations are reportedly present in 5-15% of all ovarian cancer cases.[46]

Generally speaking, the higher the number of ovulations a woman has in her lifetime the higher her chances of developing ovarian cancer. The reason for this is that when an ovary produces an egg during ovulation, the surface layer of the ovary bursts to release the egg. The surface cells then divide to repair the damage. The more eggs the ovaries produce during your lifetime, the more cells need to divide and hence the higher the chance that damage will occur that could lead to cancer. According to Cancer Research UK,[47] and other sources, the risk of ovarian cancer may also be increased by:

- getting older;
- being infertile or never giving birth;
- having had a previous breast cancer (as this may suggest the presence of a BRCA mutation);
- being overweight;
- being tall;
- having endometriosis;

- a family history of ovarian cancer;
- smoking;
- HRT (oestrogen only);
- fertility treatment.

Factors which may reduce the risk of developing ovarian cancer include having children (parity), breastfeeding, taking the contraceptive pill, having tubal ligation (having ones 'tubes tied' to prevent pregnancy) and having a hysterectomy.[47] This is most likely because these factors may be linked to less frequent ovulation.

Parity – the number of times that a woman has given birth – has been found to decrease the risk of ovarian cancer in the general population. Similar to the general population, pregnancy protects against ovarian cancer in BRCA1 mutation carriers;[19, 48] however, data regarding this association in BRCA2 mutation carriers are not definitive. One study reported a significant 44% reduction in the risk of ovarian cancer in BRCA1 mutation carriers who had given birth one or more times (are 'parous'); however, parity was associated with an increased risk of ovarian cancer in BRCA2 carriers.[19, 49]

A further study found that more full-term pregnancies among parous BRCA1 mutation carriers were associated with a reduced risk of ovarian cancer. However, the number of ovarian cancer cases in BRCA2 mutation carriers in their report was too small to provide definitive conclusions for this group of carriers.[19, 50]

The effect, if any, of **long-term breastfeeding** on ovarian cancer is unclear. For BRCA1 mutation carriers, evidence suggests that breastfeeding may be protective for ovarian cancer, but the results are not conclusive.[19, 49] However, a study published in 2009 found no significant evidence that breastfeeding was protective for ovarian cancer in BRCA1/2 mutation carriers.[50]

The use of **oral contraceptives** is associated with a reduction in ovarian cancer risk in the general population.[51] Evidence suggests that the longer women have used oral contraceptives, the greater the reduction in ovarian cancer risk. This reduction in risk has been shown to persist for more than 30 years after oral contraceptive use has ceased. According to investigators, oral contraceptives may have already prevented some 200,000 ovarian cancers and 100,000 deaths from the disease; over the next few decades the number of cancers prevented will rise to at least 30,000 per year.[51] Evidence also supports oral contraceptives being protective among BRCA1/BRCA2 mutation carriers. A meta-analysis of 18 studies including 13,627 BRCA mutation carriers reported a significantly reduced risk of ovarian cancer associated with oral contraceptive use. Specifically, the use of oral contraceptives was associated with a 50% reduced risk of ovarian cancer in BRCA1/2 carriers.[24]

Symptoms of ovarian cancer

As the symptoms of ovarian cancer can be similar to those of other conditions, it is a difficult condition to recognise. However, there are early symptoms to look out for and these may include:

- persistent bloating;
- feeling full (early satiety) and/or loss of appetite;
- pelvic or abdominal pain;
- increased urinary urgency and/or frequency;
- weight loss;
- fatigue;
- changes in bowel habit (diarrhoea or constipation, or fluctuating between the two).

It's important to see your family doctor if you experience these symptoms, particularly if they persist over a long period of time. Any woman of 50 or over who is experiencing symptoms that suggest irritable bowel syndrome (IBS) should seek medical advice as IBS rarely presents for the first time in women of this age and this is the most common wrong diagnosis for ovarian cancer.

Your family doctor may perform an internal examination to check for any masses and will also ask about your general health. A blood test to measure the levels of 'CA-125' may also be carried out. If this is raised it could be a sign of ovarian cancer and an ultrasound scan may be necessary.

If ovarian cancer is confirmed, the main treatments are surgery and chemotherapy. Almost all women with ovarian cancer will need surgery, although some women will be treated by chemotherapy alone. For some women with very early stage ovarian cancer, surgery may be the only treatment needed. However, given that the majority of women with ovarian cancer are diagnosed with advanced disease, many will have a combination of both surgery and chemotherapy. Such women may have chemotherapy after surgery, or both before and after.

Ovarian cancer in BRCA mutation carriers

In the general population, more than 90% of ovarian cancers start in the cells that cover the surface of the ovary (the epithelium) and are called epithelial ovarian cancers. In BRCA1/BRCA2-associated ovarian cancer, patients are typically diagnosed with this type of ovarian cancer. As a result, patients in the UK who are diagnosed with this cancer may now be offered BRCA gene testing to determine whether or not they carry a harmful mutation in these genes.[52]

There are various types of epithelial ovarian cancer but the most common type, and that typically seen in BRCA mutation carriers, is 'serous epithelial ovarian cancer'. The vast majority of ovarian cancers associated with BRCA gene mutations are reportedly high-grade and advanced-stage serous cancers. More specifically, over 70% of ovarian cancers in BRCA1 and BRCA2 mutation carriers are grade 3 serous cancers.[53] However, please note that borderline ovarian tumours, which are another type of epithelial ovarian tumour, are not associated with BRCA gene mutations.

When compared with sporadic ovarian cancer cases, women with BRCA-associated ovarian cancer tend to be diagnosed at a younger age. Furthermore, evidence suggests that ovarian cancer in BRCA1 mutation carriers tends to occur at a younger age than in BRCA2 mutation carriers.[54] Evidence also suggests that ovarian cancer patients carrying BRCA gene mutations have an improved chance of survival in comparison with sporadic cases. An analysis of 26 studies published in 2012 which explored survival differences between BRCA mutation carriers and non-carriers showed a more favourable prognosis (outcome) in carriers than non-carriers, with BRCA2 mutation carriers having the best prognosis.[55]

In addition to the risk for ovarian cancer, BRCA mutation carriers are also at slightly increased risk of developing other related cancers, such as fallopian tube cancer and primary peritoneal cancer (PPC).

Fallopian tube cancer

The fallopian tubes are the tubes that transport a woman's eggs from her ovaries to her uterus (womb) each month, where they are either fertilised by sperm or discarded during menstruation (see Figure 14).

Cancer of the fallopian tubes is very rare and the symptoms are similar to those of ovarian cancer. It is usually misdiagnosed as ovarian cancer, abscess or ectopic pregnancy. In the general population, the lifetime risk of developing fallopian tube cancer is 0.025%, or one in 4000 women.[56] While BRCA mutation carriers are at increased risk of developing fallopian tube cancer compared with women in the general population, the absolute risk is relatively low. According to a study published in 2003, the lifetime risk for fallopian tube cancer in BRCA mutation carriers is only 0.6%.[57]

Evidence suggests that ovarian cancer may actually begin in

the distal fallopian tube (the part of the tube closest to the ovary) and later spread to the ovary rather than having originated on the surface of the ovary itself. A study published in 2007, which aimed to review the frequency and location of malignancies detected after risk-reducing salpingo-oophorectomy in women with BRCA mutations, reported that 6% of these women had cancer at the time of risk-reducing surgery and that all of these women had cancer in the distal end of their fallopian tubes.[58] Because some ovarian cancers may start in this way, removal of both fallopian tubes in addition to the ovaries is recommended during risk-reducing surgery in high-risk women. However, even after women have undergone a bilateral salpingo-oophorectomy a small amount of the fallopian tube remains in the uterine wall and there may, therefore, be a theoretical residual risk of fallopian tube cancer.

Fallopian tube cancer in BRCA mutation carriers

In the general population, more than 95% of fallopian tube cancers start in the epithelial cells which form the surface of the fallopian tubes; they are called 'serous adenocarcinomas'.[59] In BRCA-associated fallopian tube cancer, patients are typically diagnosed with advanced-stage, high-grade, serous fallopian tube cancers. Evidence suggests that patients with BRCA-associated fallopian tube cancer are diagnosed at a younger age and have improved survival compared with patients without a BRCA gene mutation.[60]

Similarly to ovarian cancer, if detected early, fallopian tube cancer can often be successfully treated and survival is very high. At its earliest stage, where the cancer is only in the lining of the fallopian tube, the five-year survival rate is 90%, but as the cancer spreads, the survival rate decreases.[61]

Also similarly to ovarian cancer, fallopian tube cancer often produces chemicals that can be detected using a CA-125 blood test. The treatment is similar to that for ovarian cancer and may include a combination of both surgery and chemotherapy.

Primary peritoneal cancer

The peritoneum is a layer of thin tissue that lines the abdomen and covers all of the organs within it, such as the liver, bowel and stomach. Its function is to protect the organs and to act as a barrier to infection.

Primary peritoneal cancer (PPC) is a rare cancer of the peritoneum; it's very similar to epithelial ovarian cancer because the lining of the abdomen and the surface of the ovary come from the same tissue when we develop from embryos in the womb. There is a fashionable theory that all ovarian and primary peritoneal cancer is really fallopian tube cancer. However, many doctors do not believe this is true as women can still get PPC after hysterectomy with salpingo-oophorectomy and, therefore, this residual tube can't be blamed for all such cases.

Primary peritoneal cancer can be very unclear and difficult to spot, especially when it is in its early stages, but the symptoms are the same as those seen in ovarian cancer. If primary peritoneal cancer is suspected, a pelvic examination, ultrasound and CA-125 blood test may be performed.

BRCA gene mutation carriers, and in particular BRCA1 mutation carriers, are at a higher risk of developing primary peritoneal cancer than women in the general population, but the absolute risk is low. According to a study published in 2003, the lifetime risk for PPC in BRCA mutation carriers is 1.3%.[57] Currently in the UK, however, there are neither guidelines nor screening available for monitoring BRCA mutation carriers for primary peritoneal cancer.

Even after a BRCA carrier has undergone risk-reducing salpingo-oophorectomy, a small risk of primary peritoneal cancer remains because the peritoneum is made up of the same type of cells as parts of the ovary. A further study published in 2005 calculated a 3.5% lifetime risk for all mutation carriers and a 3.9% lifetime risk for BRCA1 mutation carriers through 20 years of follow-up after risk-reducing oophorectomy. Within this study, all five cases of PPC were serous carcinomas and all occurred in BRCA1 mutation carriers.[62]

Some people question whether peritoneal washing – a procedure in which the pelvis is bathed in fluid which is then collected to look for cancer cells in the peritoneum – should be performed during a risk-reducing salpingo-oophorectomy (RRSO) to determine whether or not PPC may be present. Peritoneal washes are routinely done to stage abdominal and pelvic tumours, but the role of peritoneal washings during risk-reducing surgery at this time is unclear. A study published in 2006 reported mesothelial atypia – abnormal-looking meso-thelial cells which make up the peritoneum – in 11% of patients who had peritoneal washings performed at the time of RRSO, but none of these patients later went on to develop perito-neal carcinoma.[63] According to investigators, the link between mesothelial atypia and BRCA gene mutations, and the need to perform peritoneal washings in this setting, are both yet to be de-termined. Similarly, a further study published in 2010 also found that none of the patients who had positive peritoneal washings went on to develop primary peritoneal cancer or ovarian cancer during follow-up. Based on this evidence, researchers suggest that peritoneal washing during salpingo-oophorectomy is of limited value and should not be practised routinely.[64] Currently in the UK, peritoneal washing is not routinely performed during risk-reducing surgery unless evidence of a pelvic or abdominal cancer is found. However, the protocol for risk-reducing oopho-rectomy for high-risk women in the US includes performing a peritoneal wash.[65]

9.
Uterine cancer and BRCA mutations – is there a link?

Uterine (womb) cancer is rare, but it is the most commonly occurring cancer of the female reproductive system, with most cases being diagnosed in women between the ages of 40 and 74 who have been through the menopause.[66] The exact causes of uterine cancer are unknown, but risk increases with age, exposure to oestrogen, being overweight, the use of tamoxifen and endometrial hyperplasia, among others.[66]

The vast majority of uterine cancers begin in the cells that make up the lining of the womb, known as the endometrium, which is why cancer of the uterus is often called endometrial cancer. In the general population, the majority of these tumours are low-grade, stage 1 endometrial cancers which have an excellent prognosis and most women with early-stage disease can anticipate cure with surgery alone.[67] However, there is a rare and aggressive form of uterine cancer that is not the usual highly curable endometrial cancer but a more aggressive type called 'uterine serous carcinoma' (USC), also known as 'uterine papillary serous carcinoma' (UPSC). Under the microscope, this type of uterine cancer resembles the fallopian tube cancers and ovarian cancers seen in female BRCA mutation carriers. It is often diagnosed at an advanced-stage 4 and results in a poor prognosis, which is comparable to serous cancer of the ovary.[68]

In the UK, the received wisdom is that uterine cancer is not associated with BRCA gene mutations, but, while there is a large amount of research suggesting that women with BRCA mutations are at risk of developing ovarian and fallopian tube cancers, there have only been a few studies published in relation to uterine cancer among BRCA mutation carriers and, despite this research, the effect remains unclear.

A study published in 2000 found no evidence of a BRCA1 or BRCA2 mutation in 56 patients with uterine papillary serous carcinoma (UPSC); however, a high proportion of patients with UPSC were found to have a personal history of breast cancer or a close family member with breast cancer. Researchers concluded that BRCA mutations do not appear to increase the risk of UPSC and suggested that the observed association between UPSC and breast cancer may be due to the presence of mutations in other genes.[69] Similarly, a further study published in 2001 also found no evidence of BRCA mutations in 17 UPSC patients, suggesting that the lifetime risk for uterine cancer is not increased for individuals with a BRCA gene mutation.[70]

With regard to the evidence which may suggest a link, a study published in 2002, which aimed to evaluate the risks of other cancers in BRCA1 mutation carriers only, found a statistically significant increased risk for cancer of the uterus and cervix, among others, compared with women in the general population.[71] A more recent study published in 2013 suggested that the increased risk for uterine cancer in BRCA1 mutation carriers is, however, predominantly associated with a history of tamoxifen use.[72] Therefore, this finding highlights the importance of discussing the option of hysterectomy with your gynaecologist if tamoxifen use is to be considered.

Furthermore, evidence suggests that BRCA1 mutation carriers may be at slightly increased risk of developing the rare and aggressive form of uterine cancer mentioned above – USC. A study presented at the Society of Gynecologic Oncology 2014 annual conference followed 525 BRCA mutation carriers who had undergone a BSO (bilateral salpingo-oophorectomy) and their uterus remained intact. During the follow-up of up to 17 years, four women with BRCA1 mutations were diagnosed with aggressive uterine cancer. This represented a significant increase when compared with the general population; two of the women had used tamoxifen, while the other two had not.[73]

A study published in 2010 which aimed to determine the incidence of the three mutations common in Ashkenazi Jewish patients among patients with USC found a high rate of BRCA mutations, as well as a high rate of personal and familial cancer histories, suggesting that this aggressive type of uterine cancer may be associated with BRCA gene mutations.[68] However, the link between uterine cancer and BRCA gene mutations may only be linked to certain BRCA1 mutations and not all those that have been identified.

In a study published in 2016, researchers looked at data for more than 1000 women who tested positive for either the BRCA1 or BRCA2 mutation who had undergone risk-reducing surgery to remove their ovaries and fallopian tubes. Over a follow-up period of between seven and 13 years, eight of the women developed uterine cancer, including five who developed serous/ serous-like uterine carcinoma. Researchers concluded that the risk for serous/serous-like endometrial carcinoma was increased in women with BRCA1 mutations.[74] Furthermore, using this data, researchers calculated the risk of a BRCA1 mutation carrier developing this aggressive form of uterine cancer after undergoing RRSO at the age of 45 to be between 2.6 and 4.7% (up to the age of 70).

In summary, there are studies which have failed to find a link between uterine cancer and BRCA gene mutations, and others which suggest that there may be a link between BRCA1 mutations and uterine serous carcinoma. However, the evidence so far suggests that BRCA2 mutation carriers may not be at increased risk for uterine cancer.

Clarification of this issue is necessary because, while the serous/serous-like endometrial cancer accounts for only about 10% of uterine cancer cases, it accounts for more than 40% of deaths due to the disease.[75] At the present time, however, there is simply not enough evidence to support a need for managing the risk for uterine cancer in BRCA mutation carriers.

It may be that women who choose to undergo removal of their ovaries and tubes may also wish to eliminate uterine and cervical cancer risks by opting for a total abdominal hysterectomy at the same time. Furthermore, for those women with existing gynaecologic conditions, a hysterectomy may be advisable and this possibility should be discussed with a gynaecologist.

10.
Prostate cancer

The male reproductive system includes a small gland about the size of a walnut called the prostate gland. It sits below the bladder and surrounds the urethra – the tube men urinate and ejaculate through (see Figure 15). The main role of the prostate gland is to produce prostate fluid, a thick clear fluid that is an important part of semen.

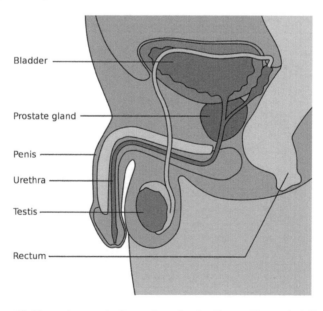

Bladder

Prostate gland

Penis

Urethra

Testis

Rectum

Figure 15: The male reproductive system showing the position and relative size of the healthy prostate gland

Prostate cancer is the second most common cancer, after lung cancer, in men worldwide[76] and it is the second leading cause of death from cancer in men in the US.[77]

In the UK, prostate cancer is the most common cancer in men and over 46,000 men are diagnosed with the disease every year. It is estimated that about one in eight men in the general UK population will be diagnosed with prostate cancer at some point in their lives.[78] Although survival rates have dramatically improved in recent years, the disease still claims nearly 11,000 lives each year.[79]

Very little is known about the causes of prostate cancer but age, being of black race and family history are known to be major risk factors for developing the disease. Specifically, men with BRCA1 and BRCA2 gene mutations have an increased risk of prostate cancer.

Prostate cancer develops mainly in older men and it is rarely diagnosed in men under the age of 45. The incidence of this disease rises rapidly with age and, globally, three-quarters of cases occur in men over the age of 65. As the world's population ages, prostate cancer is set to become an increasingly important health problem.[79]

As described earlier, for BRCA1 mutation carriers, the lifetime risk of developing prostate cancer is approximately 10% which is similar to the risk within the general population. However, for BRCA2 mutation carriers, the lifetime risk is 20-25%, which is considerably higher.[12] Evidence consistently indicates that BRCA2 carriers are more likely to develop prostate cancer at a younger age with more aggressive forms of the disease. Furthermore, in BRCA2 mutation carriers the disease has often spread by the time of diagnosis and the mortality rate is higher than for non-carriers.[80, 81, 82, 83, 84, 85]

While there is debate about whether there is an increased risk of prostate cancer for BRCA1 mutation carriers, there is increasing evidence that those BRCA1 mutation carriers who develop prostate cancer are also more likely to develop more aggressive forms of the disease.[80, 82]

Symptoms of prostate cancer

Prostate cancer does not normally cause symptoms until the cancer has grown large enough to put pressure on the urethra. This normally results in problems associated with urination. Therefore, symptoms can include:

- needing to urinate more frequently, often during the night;
- needing to rush to the toilet;
- difficulty in starting to pee (hesitancy);
- straining or taking a long time while urinating;
- weak flow when urinating;
- feeling that the bladder has not emptied fully.

However, these symptoms can be mild and happen over many years and may be a sign of a benign prostate problem, rather than prostate cancer.

For some men the first symptoms of prostate cancer may not occur until the cancer has reached a more advanced stage, when the cancer has spread into other organs of the body, such as the bones. These symptoms may include bone and back pain, a loss of appetite and unexplained weight loss. It's important to see a doctor if experiencing these symptoms, particularly if they persist over a long period of time.

The doctor may take a blood test to check the levels of a protein called 'prostate specific antigen' (PSA) in the blood. PSA is a protein which is produced by the cells of the prostate and is often elevated in men with prostate cancer. However, it can also be elevated in benign conditions, such as benign prostatic hyperplasia (enlargement of the prostate) and in individuals who have a urinary tract infection. The doctor may also do an examination of the prostate gland, known as a digital rectal examination, which involves a finger being inserted into the rectum to feel for any signs of prostate cancer, such as a hard and bumpy prostate.

Types of prostate cancer in BRCA mutation carriers

In the general population, more than 90% of prostate cancers are a type known as 'acinar adenocarcinoma' (pronounced ass-in-ar ad-en-oh-car-sin-oh-ma). Many of these cancers grow extremely slowly and are not likely to spread. However, there are rarer types of prostate cancer which can be more aggressive. One of these rare and aggressive cancers, ductal adenocarcinoma, is the type typically diagnosed in BRCA mutation carriers. It starts in the cells that line the ducts (tubes) of the prostate gland and tends to grow and spread more quickly.

Men who are diagnosed with ductal adenocarcinoma are more likely to require radical treatment, including surgery to remove the prostate (known as a 'prostatectomy') or radical radiotherapy. Even with radical treatment, men with ductal adenocarcinoma have a higher likelihood of residual disease requiring additional treatment, including chemotherapy.

Men, who have their prostate removed, may experience the following:
- **erectile dysfunction** – difficulty with getting or keeping an erection can be caused by damage to the nerves during surgery;
- **infertility** – removing the prostate gland makes it impossible for men to ejaculate;
- **urinary incontinence** – a problem controlling the bladder. Most men have some incontinence straight after their operation but this usually goes away with time.

11.
Other BRCA-associated cancers

As more research is carried out into hereditary breast and ovarian cancer, more is being learnt about additional cancers associated with BRCA gene mutations, including, for example, pancreatic cancer and melanoma.

This section looks briefly at these additional cancers, and provides statistics on the level of risk for BRCA mutation carriers where possible. However, for further information, please consult with a cancer genetics expert who will know the most up-to-date risk information and will be able to provide advice on the options for risk management.

Pancreatic cancer

The pancreas is an organ which sits in the abdomen, behind the stomach and intestines. It produces important hormones, such as insulin, which help to regulate blood sugar levels, and it also produces pancreatic juice which is essential for the digestion of proteins, carbohydrates and fats.

Pancreatic cancer can affect people of any age, but it mainly affects people between the ages of 50 and 80 years. Almost 50% of people diagnosed with cancer of the pancreas are aged 75 or over.[86]

The main risk factors[87] for pancreatic cancer include:

- increasing age;
- smoking;
- being overweight;
- a family history of pancreatic cancer;
- chronic pancreatitis (long-term inflammation of the pancreas);
- diabetes.

Symptoms and diagnosis of pancreatic cancer

Like ovarian cancer, pancreatic cancer tends not to produce symptoms in the early, treatable stages, unless the cancer blocks bile outflow from the liver and causes jaundice (yellowing of the skin and whites of the eyes). Other symptoms may include:

- pain in the stomach area or back;
- bowel disturbances;
- unexplained weight loss.

Even when suspected, pancreatic cancer can be challenging to diagnose. The pancreas may appear normal on ultrasound or CT scan and require 'blind' samples to be taken. A blind sample is when the pancreas is biopsied in an area where it is thought that the cancer is present, but at the time of biopsy a clear mass is not visualised by scanning. In other circumstances the organ may appear very abnormal due to scarring, for instance due to pancreatic inflammation, making it impossible to ascertain what is 'normal' or 'abnormal'. In both of these scenarios, a negative result does not exclude cancer and a pragmatic 'watch and wait' approach is often taken, with follow-up scans arranged after a number of months have passed.

While pancreatic cancer survival rates have been improving from decade to decade, the disease is still considered largely incurable for the reasons listed above. Out of 20 common cancers in England and Wales, 10-year survival for pancreatic cancer ranks lowest overall.[88] According to the American Cancer Society, for all stages of pancreatic cancer combined, the one-year relative survival rate is 20%, and the five-year rate is 6%. These low survival rates can be explained by the fact that pancreatic cancer is often diagnosed at a late stage, with fewer than 20% of patients' tumours being confined to the pancreas at the time of diagnosis and, in most cases, the cancer has already progressed to the point where surgical removal is impossible.[89]

BRCA mutation carriers and screening

Pancreatic cancer is rare, with individuals in the general population having a lifetime risk of 1.4%.[90] BRCA mutation carriers appear to be at increased risk of developing this cancer, particularly if a first-degree relative (i.e. a parent, sibling or child) is diagnosed with it. The risk for BRCA2 mutation carriers is estimated to be up to 3.5 times greater than the general population, rising to a six-fold increase when a first-degree relative has pancreatic cancer. In addition, pancreatic cancer associated with a BRCA2 gene mutation tends to appear about a decade earlier than sporadic disease.[91, 92] The risk for BRCA1 mutation carriers is less well defined than for BRCA2 mutation carriers.[93, 94]

Screening for pancreatic cancer is not widely recommended, due to the low rate of disease in the general population and lack of a good screening test; however, a group of international experts agree that high-risk individuals, in whom the lifetime risk of pancreatic cancer exceeds 5%, should undergo screening.[94] As the risk for carriers of BRCA1 mutations is not well defined, screening is not recommended. However, screening is recommended for BRCA2 mutation carriers with a first-degree relative (i.e. a parent, sibling or child) with pancreatic cancer.[95]

The consensus of expert opinions was not able to give a recommendation on the age when high-risk individuals should first undergo screening, but repeated imaging was recommended every 12 months (although there is very limited evidence to support this strategy).

The recommended screening tools include:

- magnetic resonance imaging (MRI);
- endoscopic ultrasound (EUS) – this is a test using an endoscope with a tiny ultrasound probe attached.

Research is on-going looking for blood markers of pancreatic cancer; however, there is currently no effective screening available. CA 19-9 is a blood marker used to monitor response to chemotherapy in patients with diagnosed pancreatic cancer, but it is of no value as a screening test as it can be normal in pancreatic cancer and abnormal in other conditions, such as pancreatitis.

Any individual with a BRCA gene mutation, and particularly a BRCA2 gene mutation, who has a family history of pancreatic cancer, should consult their genetics specialist to determine risk before discussing the pros and cons of undergoing annual screening for pancreatic cancer with a pancreas specialist.

Melanoma

Melanoma is the most dangerous form of skin cancer. It is estimated that more than 2000 people in Britain and 10,000 people in the US die from the disease each year.[96, 97] If melanoma is recognised and treated early, it is almost always curable, but, if it is not, the cancer can advance and spread to other parts of the body, where it becomes hard to treat and can be fatal.

Melanoma may arise in the skin (cutaneous melanoma) and also in the eye (uveal melanoma). It is thought to be caused mainly by intense UV exposure, especially in those who are genetically predisposed to the disease.[97] According to Cancer Research UK, skin melanoma is on the rise, with around 13,300 people being diagnosed with skin melanoma each year, compared with around 1800 in the mid-1970s. The increase is thought to be partly due to the rising popularity of package holidays and the use of sun beds.[98]

Research evaluating the association between BRCA1/2 mutations and skin cancer is limited and has produced inconsistent results. However, a review of this literature published in 2015 reported that BRCA2 may be associated with melanoma, but no studies have shown a statistically significant risk of melanoma in BRCA1 mutation carriers.[99] Evidence suggests that BRCA2 mutation carriers have approximately double to triple the risk of melanoma compared with those without a BRCA2 gene mutation. Specifically, it has been reported that BRCA2 mutation carriers have 2.58 times greater risk than non-carriers of developing melanoma.[100]

Currently in the UK, there is insufficient evidence to warrant increased skin cancer surveillance among BRCA mutation carriers. However, if there is a high incidence of skin melanoma in a family associated with the BRCA gene mutation, patients are increasingly being referred for screening by a dermatologist. A dermatologist can then use a specialised magnification instrument, called a dermatoscope, to observe moles for any signs of cancer. Full-body photography may also be used to track mole changes over a period of time.

Nonetheless, it is very important for a BRCA1/2 mutation carrier to be aware of the potential for increased risk of melanoma, to regularly check for signs of cancer and also to use a high factor sunscreen.

Symptoms of melanoma

Skin cancers are found mainly on areas of the skin that are exposed to the sun – the head, face, lips, ears, neck, hands and arms – but they can occur anywhere on the body.

It is so important to detect melanoma early that physicians have developed two specific strategies for early recognition of the disease:

- The 'ugly duckling' sign: This method is based on the concept that these melanomas look different – they are 'ugly ducklings'– compared with surrounding moles. The premise is that the patient's 'normal' moles resemble each other, like siblings, while the potential melanoma is an 'outlier', a lesion that, at a given moment in time, *looks* or *feels* different from the patient's other moles or that, over time, changes differently from the patient's other moles.
- The ABCDE rule: The ABCDE rule is another guide to the usual signs of melanoma. Be on the lookout and report to a doctor any spots that have any of the following features:

  A = Asymmetry – symmetrical or asymmetrical?

  B = Border – even or uneven?

  C = Colour – one or multiple colours?

  D = Diameter – smaller or larger than ¼ inch (0.6 cm)?

  E = Evolving – changing in size, shape and/or colours?

It is important to self-examine moles on a regular basis and to recognise any changes in the skin. If there is any concern at all, advice should be sought from a doctor. This advice is important for all individuals, but for anyone with a BRCA gene mutation, and in particular a BRCA2 mutation, it is especially important to follow this advice and check your skin on a monthly basis.

Some melanomas do not fit the ABCDE rule and, therefore, any changes or new spots on your skin, or any growth that stands out, should be highlighted to a doctor. Other worrying signs that may suggest melanoma include:

- a sore that doesn't heal,
- the spread of pigment from the border of a spot into the surrounding skin,

- redness, or a new swelling beyond the border,
- itchiness, tenderness or pain and
- changes to the surface of a mole, such as scaliness, oozing, bleeding, or the appearance of a bump or nodule.

Uveal melanoma (eye cancer)

Uveal melanoma forms in the pigment cells of the uvea, which is the middle layer of the eye. While uveal melanoma is rare, it is the most common primary cancer of the eye. In the US, there are between 1200 and 1500 new cases per year, and it accounts for about 5% of all melanomas.[101] Being older and having fair skin, red or blonde hair and blue eyes may all increase the risk of melanoma of the eye.

BRCA2 mutation carriers are at increased risk of melanoma of the eye.[102] However, further research is needed in order to determine precise levels of risk among BRCA mutation carriers.

Symptoms of uveal melanoma

Eye melanoma may not cause signs and symptoms, but when they do occur, they may include:
- a growing dark spot on the iris;
- a sensation of flashing lights;
- a change in the shape of the dark circle (pupil) at the centre of the eye;
- poor or blurry vision in one eye;
- loss of peripheral vision;
- sensation of flashes and specks of dust in a person's vision (floaters).

Anyone experiencing any of these symptoms should seek advice from their doctor and/or book an eye examination with an optician. In the light of the potential risk for uveal melanoma, BRCA mutation carriers would be best advised to have an annual eye examination by a specialist, in which an optometrist will check the health of their eyes.

How to prevent skin cancer

Sunburn not only causes considerable discomfort in the short term, but is a clear sign that the DNA in the skin cells has been damaged. Over time, this damage can lead to skin cancer. While melanoma is caused mainly by intense UV exposure which frequently leads to sunburn, remember that even without burning, tanned skin is still damaged skin.[103]

To prevent skin cancer from developing and to delay skin ageing, people of all ethnicities, whether they carry a BRCA gene mutation or not, are encouraged to follow the guidance listed below[97] though a small amount of sun daily is beneficial for ensuring enough vitamin D (see page 146).

- seek the shade, especially between 10:00 am and 4:00 pm as the summer sun is most damaging to skin in the middle of the day;
- do not burn;
- avoid sun beds;
- use a sunscreen and lip balm with an SPF of 15 or higher every day (the higher the SPF, the better the protection);
- apply plenty of sunscreen to all exposed areas at least 20 minutes before going outside. Reapply every two hours or immediately after swimming or excessive sweating (even 'waterproof' sun creams should be reapplied). Sunscreens absorb ultraviolet light so that sun doesn't reach the skin, while sun blocks create a physical barrier to block UV rays;
- cover up with clothing, including a broad-brimmed

hat and UV-blocking sunglasses (this may be especially true for BRCA mutation carriers as they may be at increased risk of uveal melanoma);

- keep newborns out of the sun. Sunscreens should be used on babies over the age of six months, choosing sunscreens that are formulated for children and babies' skin, as these are less likely to cause irritation. (Remember that childhood sunburns are believed to greatly increase the risk of melanoma later in life);
- examine your skin from head to toe every month.

Research suggests that regular daily use of a sun protection factor (SPF) of 15 or above which is effective against UVA and UVB reduces the risk of developing melanoma by 50%.[104] However, an SPF of 15 only offers a very light protection; using an SPF of 30 or above would offer far better protection against skin cancer. A daily facial moisturiser of at least SPF 30 should be worn all year round, even during the autumn/winter periods. Furthermore, during intense sunshine, SPF 50 should be worn at all times, along with the other precautionary measures of wearing a hat, sunglasses and seeking the shade wherever possible.

Finally, it is important to remember that sunscreen should not be used as an excuse to stay out in the sun, but it instead offers protection when exposure is unavoidable.

Other related cancers

Other cancers have also been described in BRCA mutation carriers, including colorectal (bowel), gastric (stomach), buccal cavity (mouth), pharynx, laryngeal, oesophagus, lung, gall bladder and bile duct, bone and cervical cancer.[71, 91, 102, 105, 106, 107]

However, currently in the UK, BRCA mutation carriers are not offered surveillance for these cancers as the risks are low. The EMBRACE study being conducted in Cambridge, England, is trying to establish whether BRCA1 and BRCA2 mutations are associated with elevated risks of these and other cancers and to study the implications for screening.

For further information, please consult a cancer genetics expert who will know the most up-to-date risk information and will be able to give advice on the options for risk management.

Section IV

Managing your risk

This section covers the various ways in which a BRCA mutation carrier can manage his or her risk of developing cancer. This includes the process of referral to a specialist genetics service, BRCA gene testing and the various options available to a BRCA mutation carrier, including screening, chemoprevention and risk-reducing surgery.

Although parts of this section, such as the testing guidelines, are specific to the UK, much of what follows is likely to be relevant to all individuals seeking information about BRCA mutations.

12.
Referral to a specialist genetics service

In the UK, guidelines published by the National Institute for Health and Care Excellence (NICE) say that women should be referred to a specialist genetics service for BRCA gene testing only if they are likely to have a high risk of developing breast cancer. NICE defines a high risk as having a one in three chance at some point in the person's life, or a greater than one in 12 chance before the age of 50. Other countries have different, but similar, guidelines.

A questionnaire regarding personal and family history of cancer completed in advance of referral helps assess relative risk and eligibility for testing.

Genetic counselling

Genetic counsellors are health professionals who have been trained to provide genetic information and support; some may have a background in nursing or social work.

In the UK, genetic counselling and BRCA testing may be offered if your family includes:

- several individuals who have had breast cancer (especially at a young age);
- individuals who have had breast and ovarian cancer;
- individuals with a specific type of ovarian cancer at any age;

- Ashkenazi Jewish ancestry with a history of breast or ovarian cancer;
- a known BRCA mutation.

The affected family members must be close, blood relatives of the person requesting testing, and must all be from the same side of the family (either the mother's or the father's). In the UK, according to the NICE guideline on familial breast cancer, BRCA testing should be offered to patients who have a 10% or greater chance of having a BRCA gene mutation.

At the genetic clinic a detailed family history will be taken and the pros and cons of undergoing genetic testing discussed to help the patient decide whether to have this test and to prepare them to receive the result, which may be positive or negative. If positive, it may have implications for other blood relatives. If a person is found to carry a harmful mutation, genetic counselling will also help with deciding on screening, chemoprevention, risk-reducing surgery and other options. It is, therefore, important to receive this genetic counselling both before and after gene testing.

Because the knowledge of a mutation can cause great anxiety, genetic counsellors are trained to support patients through any emotional reactions and to be a neutral person who can help individuals come to their own decisions. Some individuals may choose not to be tested or to postpone testing until a later date, while others may choose to be tested as soon as possible.

Genetic counsellors can also guide people with known BRCA mutations towards the best family planning decisions for them, individually. Whether to have children may be a significant source of stress for women who learn of their BRCA mutation during their childbearing years. These fertility issues are often considered by young BRCA mutation carriers to be at least as important as the cancer risk and often intensify and complicate the emotional load.

Some women who know or suspect they have an increased

risk of breast cancer simply choose to go ahead and have a family as they had always planned in the hope that new treatments may be available in the future once their children are at the age of risk. However, some may decide to limit the number of children they have and some may even decide not to have any children at all, so that they do not pass on the risk. Alternatively, some may choose to have 'pre-implantation genetic diagnosis' (PGD) which enables both women and men with a BRCA mutation to avoid passing it on to their children.

Pre-implantation genetic testing is a technique which involves screening embryos that have been created through in vitro fertilisation (IVF) for a BRCA1/BRCA2 gene mutation. A woman's eggs are removed and then fertilised (in a laboratory setting) with sperm. When the embryos are only eight cells in size (very early in the development process), one cell is removed and is tested for the BRCA gene mutation. Only those embryos identified as being free of the mutation will then be implanted and, all being well, couples can have the peace of mind that their child will not carry a harmful mutation. However, this is a complex procedure with physical and emotional factors to consider before starting. Currently, in the UK, the NHS will commission three cycles of PGD for couples who carry a BRCA gene mutation and who wish to avoid the birth of an affected child. However, patients can only be referred via their genetics centre, not via their family doctor.

The BRCA1 and BRCA2 genetic test

Following consultation with a genetic counsellor, if a patient is eligible for BRCA gene testing and decides to pursue this, an appointment will be made for blood to be drawn at a convenient time. If the genetic test is for a known mutation in the family, the test results are likely to be ready approximately four weeks after the blood sample is taken. Before the blood is drawn for the test, the genetic counsellor will discuss how the patient would like to be given the results. This could be a clinic appointment or by telephone at a mutually agreed time or by writing. A follow-up consultation should also be arranged to discuss the results in more detail and if the patient is found to carry a harmful BRCA gene mutation, a personalised screening plan can be arranged.

During a genetic test, DNA is extracted from the white blood cells contained within the blood sample. The test examines the DNA code for the BRCA1 and BRCA2 genes to look for known harmful BRCA gene mutations which are likely to cause an increased risk of breast and ovarian cancer.

Genetic testing can be done for the following reasons:

1. **Diagnostic testing** is offered to women affected with breast/ovarian cancer where the personal and family history of cancer meets testing criteria. The BRCA1 and BRCA2 gene will be examined for any pathogenic (harmful) mutations. The results of this test can influence a person's choices about health care and the management of his/her cancer. The results for diagnostic testing are usually available within 12 weeks.

2. **Predictive testing** is available for families where the genetic mutation has already been found. This test will show whether someone has inherited the familial mutation. If the mutation is not present then the individual is not at increased risk of cancer. The results of this test provide information about a person's risk of developing cancer and may help with making decisions about medical care. The results for predictive testing are usually available within four weeks.

3. **Ashkenazi Jewish mutation testing** looks for the three common mutations which are responsible for 97% of BRCA mutations in Jewish families. If a person has breast/ovarian cancer and this test is normal, then it is possible to go onto full BRCA sequencing if the family history meets the NHS genetic testing criteria.

Test results

Diagnostic BRCA testing

Diagnostic testing can give several possible results: positive, negative or ambiguous/uncertain. If the test comes back as positive (meaning that a mutation has been identified in either the BRCA1 or BRCA2 gene), this will provide an explanation for that person's and family's history of breast and/or ovarian cancer.

If a test result comes back as negative, that means that the person has not been found to carry a mutation in either of the BRCA genes. However, it is possible that the person may carry a harmful BRCA gene mutation that has not yet been identified. Furthermore, it is also possible for people to have a mutation in other genes besides BRCA1 or BRCA2 which increases their cancer risk but which is not detectable by the BRCA gene test. In this case, if this person has a strong family history of breast cancer, they may still be offered the option of screening.

Finally, the genetic test may also identify 'variants of uncertain significance' (VUS), meaning that there is a variation in the BRCA1/BRCA2 genetic code that may, or may not, be harmful. Some mutations are completely harmless and, therefore, there could be changes in the DNA which show up on a genetic test that don't actually increase the risk of cancer. This is why genetic counselling is important as the genetic team have the training to interpret the results. Variants are monitored by the laboratory and, should the classification change, the laboratory notifies the clinical genetics team who then act on the information. However, in the event that this does not happen, it is good for patients to check on updates of their variants with their genetics service every couple of years.

Predictive BRCA testing

Predictive testing can give either a positive or a negative result. It is conclusive and shows if an individual has inherited the BRCA mutation or not.

As is true for both diagnostic and predictive testing, a positive test result indicates that a person has inherited a known harmful mutation in the BRCA1 or BRCA2 gene. Both men and women who inherit a harmful BRCA gene mutation have an increased risk of developing certain cancers. Furthermore, they may pass this mutation on to their sons and daughters. As previously mentioned (page 31), each child has a 50% chance of inheriting the mutation. In addition to this, if an individual learns that he/she carries a harmful mutation, this may also have important health implications for any siblings as they too will have a 50% chance of carrying the mutation. Those who test positive for a BRCA gene mutation may be referred by either their genetic counsellor or their family doctor for breast screening and they may also be referred to a gynaecological oncologist (a gynaecologist who specialises in cancer of the female reproductive system) and breast surgeon for a further discussion of the various ways to manage their cancer risk.

A negative predictive result means that the person has not been found to carry the BRCA gene mutation that has been found in other relative(s) of their family. In this case, the person will not be at a high risk of developing cancer, their risk will fall to that of the general population and they will be recommended to participate in the National Breast Screening Programme that is available to all women between the ages of 50 and 70 years.

Men with a negative test result can feel reassured to know that they have the same extremely low risk of getting male breast cancer as men in the general population and the same relatively low risk of prostate cancer.

The benefits of genetic testing for a BRCA gene mutation

There are benefits to genetic testing, regardless of whether a person receives a positive or a negative result. The potential benefits of an individual testing negative for a BRCA gene mutation may include a sense of relief regarding his/her future risk of cancer, learning that his/her children are not at risk of inheriting the family's susceptibility to cancer, and the possibility that special check-ups, tests or risk-reducing surgeries may not be needed.

However, an individual testing positive for a BRCA gene mutation can bring relief from uncertainty and allow people to make informed decisions about their future, including measures to help lower their lifetime risk of developing cancer. It is also important for these individuals to share this result with their family when they feel it is appropriate, as it may be life-saving information to other family members. Other benefits include the possibility of participating in medical research which in the future could help to reduce deaths from breast and ovarian cancer.

The drawbacks of testing for a BRCA gene mutation

While there is no risk or harm associated with genetic testing, knowledge of test results may have harmful effects on a person's emotions, social relationships, finances and medical choices.

One of the challenges that BRCA mutation carriers face is coping with the uncertainty of what the future holds, both personally and for their family. They are likely to have to make difficult, life-changing decisions about whether to have risk-reducing surgery or about which surgery to have, without the benefit of all the facts they would like. People who receive a positive test result may feel anxious, frustrated, depressed or even angry at times.

On the other hand, people who receive a negative test result may experience 'survivor guilt', caused by the knowledge that they most likely don't have an increased risk of developing cancer that affects other family members. Because genetic testing can reveal information about more than one family member, the emotions caused by test results can create tension within families. Relationships may be affected if one person has a positive test result and their relative has a negative one.

Test results can also affect personal choices, such as decisions about starting a relationship, marriage and childbearing. For example, when starting a new relationship, at what point is it best to raise the issue of a known BRCA gene mutation? In any case, the genetic counsellor is trained to help with these emotions.

What is right for you

If you are known to carry a harmful mutation, breast health specialists, genetic counsellors, gynaecologic oncologists and primary health care physicians all have an important role in helping you to come to a decision as to how you can lower your risk for both breast and ovarian cancer. Discuss each of the possible options with your family doctor and the specialists that you are referred to. Don't be afraid to seek opinions and recommendations from several professionals in the process of deciding on the best risk reduction plan for you. Also, don't be afraid to read as widely as possible on and around this topic. It may take you some time to feel that you have absorbed enough information to be confident about your decisions, but hopefully, given time, you will feel empowered to make a decision.

The next chapter (Screening, page 112) provides an overview of the various ways in which a carrier can manage his/her mutation, including screening, chemoprevention and risk-reducing surgery. There is no 'right' choice. Everyone has to decide which is best for them, and what feels like the right option for one person may not be for another. If you carry a BRCA gene mutation, it is important that you make the choice that is right for *you*.

13.
Screening

Breast screening

Screening refers to tests and examinations used to find a disease, such as cancer, in people who do not have any symptoms. The goal of screening examinations for breast cancer is to find cancer early before it starts to cause symptoms. It is important to understand that screening cannot prevent breast cancer developing, but the aim is to detect cancer at an early stage when it is more likely to be curable.

Breast cancers that are found because they are causing symptoms tend to be larger and are more likely to have already spread beyond the breast. In contrast, breast cancers found during screening are more likely to be smaller and still confined to the breast. The size of a breast cancer and how far it has spread are some of the most important factors in predicting the prognosis (outlook). It has been shown that early detection of breast cancer saves thousands of lives each year, and that many more lives could be saved if even more women and their health care providers took advantage of these tests.

Because women who carry a BRCA gene mutation have a high risk of breast cancer, it is important they have increased breast cancer screening. According to NICE's guideline on familial breast cancer, women with known BRCA1 or BRCA2 gene mutations are currently offered:

- annual MRI screening from the age of 30-40;
- annual mammography and annual MRI between the ages of 40 and 49;
- annual mammography from the age of 50 onwards.

The use of magnetic resonance imaging (MRI) is a newer form of breast screening that has been introduced for young women at increased risk of breast cancer because it is more sensitive for detecting breast cancers than mammography.[1] In the UK, men are not offered breast screening, but are informed of the signs and symptoms to look out for and are advised to raise any concerns with their family doctor.

Magnetic resonance imaging (MRI)

MRI is a type of scan that uses strong magnetic fields and radio waves to produce detailed images of the inside of the body.

During a breast MRI, the patient receives an injection of contrast material into the bloodstream, the most commonly used such contrast containing a magnetic metal called gadolinium, which ensures a clear image.

As gadolinium flows through the bloodstream and enters the magnetic field, its temperature increases slightly. (Patients will not feel this effect because the amount of the element is so small.) The signals created by the flowing gadolinium are detected by the MRI scanner and analysed by computer to create images of the breast tissue. The presence of the gadolinium in the veins highlights the circulation inside the breast and helps create a high-contrast image. Gadolinium will cool off as it exits the magnetic field and will be cleared from the body by the kidneys.

Breast lesions are usually identified because they are enhanced after the injection of this contrast agent. It is also possible to see whether the breasts are dense in pattern. Figure 16 shows invasive breast cancer scanned with MRI, which was not visible by either mammography or ultrasound. It is possible to see very clearly how the contrast agent has enhanced the image of cancerous regions of the breast.

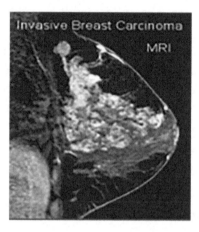

Figure 16: Breast cancer revealed on MRI through dynamic contrast enhancement

Is MRI safe?

Since a breast MRI uses an extremely low dose of gadolinium, there is very little risk of overdose or side-effects. No short-term harmful effects have been found from MRI scans. The use of magnetic fields is not thought to be harmful; however, long-term side-effects are unknown. There is a very small risk from the effects of the contrast material, but this is extremely rare. These reactions are usually mild and may include itchy skin or pain at the injection site.

However, one drawback of MRI screening is that there is a higher recall rate to investigate abnormalities that may not be cancer, compared with mammography.[2]

Mammography

Mammography is a specific type of breast imaging that uses low-dose X-rays to detect cancer early. A screening mammogram is used to look for signs of breast cancer when you do not have any symptoms or problems.

A mammogram looks only at breast tissue and the machine produces an X-ray image at lower doses than a usual X-ray machine. Because these X-rays do not go through tissue easily, the machine has two plates that compress or flatten the breast to spread the tissue apart; this gives a better picture and uses less radiation. The latest advance in mammography, known as tomosynthesis or digital tomosynthesis, is a special kind of mammogram that produces a three-dimensional image of the breast by using several low dose X-rays obtained at different angles. The breast is positioned the same way it is in a standard mammogram, but only a little pressure is applied – just enough to keep the breast in a stable position during the procedure. Early research suggests that tomosynthesis should give a more accurate and detailed picture of the breast than standard mammograms[3] and it should help to make breast screening more comfortable.

Mammograms may increase the chance of detecting breast cancer at an early stage, when it may have a better chance of being treated successfully. If a woman over 50 has breast cancer there is about 85% chance that mammography will detect it. However, the sensitivity of mammography in young BRCA carriers (aged 35-49) has been demonstrated to be only around 40%.[2] For this reason, young BRCA mutation carriers are recommended to have annual MRI screening as this form of screening is more sensitive for detecting breast cancer,[1] and this low level of sensitivity with mammography is also one of the reasons that women are recommended to have annual mammography rather than every two or three years.[2]

A mammogram can often detect cancer in its early stages, even before a lump can be felt, and it is at this point that treatment may have the most successful outcome. Mammograms can't prove that an abnormal area is cancer, but they can give information that shows whether more testing is needed. The two main types of breast changes found with a mammogram are calcifications and masses. Calcifications are tiny mineral deposits within the breast tissue, which look like small white spots on the pictures. They may or may not be caused by cancer. A mass, which may or may not have calcifications, is another important change seen on mammograms. Masses can be many things, including cysts (fluid-filled sacs) and non-cancerous solid tumours, but they could also be cancer. Any mass that's not clearly a simple fluid-filled cyst usually needs to be biopsied to see if cancer cells are present.

Having your older mammograms available for the radiologist is very important. They can help to show if a mass or calcification has changed over time, which could affect whether a biopsy is needed.

After the mammogram, the doctor can look at the pictures on a computer screen and adjust the size, brightness or contrast to see certain areas more clearly. Digital images can also be sent electronically to another site for other breast specialists to see.

Is mammography safe?

As mammograms use X-rays and radiation can lead to cancer, people who have mammograms are at risk, albeit a low risk, of developing radiation-associated breast cancer. This is of particular concern with women who carry a BRCA gene mutation because a mutated BRCA gene seems to lose its ability to repair DNA which can be caused by exposure to radiation, thereby possibly further increasing a woman's likelihood of developing breast cancer.

In addition to extending some lives by early detection and treatment, there are concerns over missed diagnoses and over-diagnosis. Over-diagnosis refers to the diagnosis and treatment of breast cancer that would never have made a woman ill in her lifetime – she would never have known about it if she had not been screened. Unfortunately, it is very difficult for doctors to know whether a particular cancer would lead to death or would have remained undetected for the rest of the woman's life.[4]

Breast density

Breasts are said to be dense if they have a lot of fibro-glandular tissue and not much fat. The fibro-glandular breast tissue is the network of milk glands and ducts designed to produce and transport milk to the nipple for breastfeeding. Fibrous tissue, also known as connective tissue, supports the breasts and holds everything in place.

Breast density can be inherited so, if the patient's mother has dense breasts, it's likely she will, too. It is also related to body fat composition; overweight women's breasts will not be as dense as slim women's. Dense breasts are very common and are not abnormal. Approximately half of all women over 40 years old have dense breasts.[5] Unfortunately, a woman often does not know if she has dense breast tissue – it is not the same as 'lumpy' breasts. Breast density can only be determined by the appearance of the breast on mammogram, or MRI, and not by feel. The denser a woman's breast tissue is, the more 'white' the breast will appear on a mammogram, whereas women with mostly fatty breasts will have a mammogram that appears darker.

The BI-RADS classification system identifies four levels of breast density. Figure 17 shows these levels.[6]

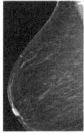 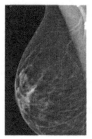 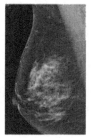 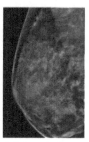

| 1. Almost entirely fatty | 2. Scattered areas of fibroglandular density | 3. Heterogeneously dense | 4. Extremely dense |

Figure 17: Levels of breast density

Dense breasts can make it harder for mammograms to detect breast cancer. On mammograms, dense breast tissue looks white, and breast tumours also look white. So, the dense tissue can hide tumours. As a result, mammograms can be less accurate in detecting tumours in women with dense breasts.[7] In general, approximately 10-20% of breast cancers are missed by standard mammography and that percentage can approach 40-50% in women with dense breast tissue.[8] Having dense breast tissue might increase the risk of getting breast cancer, compared with women with less dense breast tissue. In fact, one of the strongest known risk factors for breast cancer is high breast density. Research has shown that women with dense breast tissue in 75% or more of their breasts have a four to six times greater risk of breast cancer than women with little or no dense breast tissue.[9] However, evidence suggests that increased breast density is not associated with higher breast cancer incidence in women with BRCA gene mutations.[10, 11]

It is unclear at this time why dense breast tissue is linked with breast cancer risk, but there are a couple of possible explanations. Firstly, the development of atypical ductal hyperplasia is more likely in an 'elevated growth' environment. Secondly, a woman may have naturally overactive aromatase, which increases oestrogen production within the breast, and may stimulate the growth of tumour cells.[12]

Currently, in the UK, it is not mandatory for patients to be informed of their breast density classification and often they will, therefore, be unaware of their breast density. However, in the US, breast density notification laws have now been put into effect in many states requiring patients to be notified of their breast density.[13]

What is the cause of dense breasts?

Breast density changes throughout a woman's life and typically decreases with age. Breast density is also known to be influenced by other factors such as genetics, body mass index, monthly hormonal cycles, age at first childbirth and use of postmenopausal hormone replacement therapy (HRT).

Breast density decreases somewhat with each pregnancy; the more children a woman has given birth to, the less dense her breasts tend to be. Similarly, the more children a woman has given birth to, the lower her risk of breast cancer. With regard to body mass index (BMI), women who are obese with a high BMI tend to have a high abundance of fat within their breast tissue. High levels of fat within the breasts, relative to the amount of fibro-glandular breast tissue, would lead to a low breast density.

It is generally accepted that oestrogen levels are a major cause of dense breasts, particularly since premenopausal women (who have higher levels of oestrogen) are more likely to have dense breasts than postmenopausal women.[14] In addition, it seems that breast density changes during the menstrual cycle, becoming denser in the latter part of the cycle in response to oestrogen exposure. Since postmenopausal hormone therapy can increase breast density,[14] and because HRT is in itself a risk factor for breast cancer, women with dense breasts may want to explore other options to manage menopausal symptoms.

Breast self-examination

Breast self-examination was originally proposed and implemented on the assumption that it would increase detection of the disease at an earlier stage, in which case treatment would be more effective and, theoretically, improve survival. Early diagnosis remains an important strategy, particularly in low- and middle-income countries where the disease is more commonly diagnosed in late stages and resources are very limited.

There is no evidence on the effect of screening through breast self-examination (BSE). However, the practice of BSE has been seen to empower women, helping them to take responsibility for their own health. Therefore, BSE is recommended for raising awareness among women at risk rather than as a recommended screening method.

It is important for all women to examine their breasts on a regular basis (once a month) and to do so at around the same time in the cycle each month as the breasts will feel different at different parts of a woman's cycle. For example, at ovulation time and prior to menstruation, there is more fluid retention in the breast tissue making it feel lumpier, fuller and more sensitive. Therefore, it is best not routinely to do this examination around ovulation time and prior to menstruation.

If you are aware that you carry a BRCA gene mutation, or if there is a strong family history of breast cancer, then it is absolutely vital that you examine your breasts on a regular basis. Men who have a strong family history of breast cancer, or who carry a BRCA gene mutation, and especially a BRCA2 mutation, may also benefit from breast self-examinations.

How to do a breast self-examination
1.   Begin by looking at your breasts in the mirror with your shoulders straight and your arms on your hips. You should look out for breasts that are:
     •   their usual size, shape, and colour;
     •   evenly shaped without visible distortion or swelling.

2. If you see any areas of dimpling, puckering or bulging of the skin, a nipple that has changed position or an inverted nipple (pushed inward instead of sticking out) or redness, soreness, rash or swelling, bring this to your doctor's attention.

3. Now, raise your arms and look for the same changes. Look for any signs of fluid coming out of one or both nipples (this may be a watery, milky, yellow fluid or blood).

4. Next, lay down wherever is comfortable. Use your right hand to feel your left breast and then your left hand to feel your right breast. Use a firm, smooth touch with the first few finger pads of your hand, keeping the fingers flat and together. Use a small, circular motion. Make sure you examine the entire breast from top to bottom, side to side – from your collarbone to the top of your abdomen, and from your armpit to your cleavage. (Remember that breast tissue can sometimes extend to the collarbone and armpit.)

5. Next, stand up and check your breasts in this position. It is vital to check your breasts when standing and lying down, as some women have been able to feel a lump lying down that they were unable to feel when standing, and vice versa. Many women find that the easiest way to feel their breasts is when their skin is wet and slippery, so they like to do this step in the shower. Examine your entire breast, using the same hand movements described in step 4.

Follow a set pattern to be sure that you cover the whole breast. You can begin at the nipple, moving in larger and larger circles until you reach the outer edge of the breast. You can also move your fingers up and down vertically, in rows, if you prefer. Be sure to feel all the tissue from the front to the back of your breasts: for the skin and tissue just beneath, use light pressure;

use medium pressure for tissue in the middle of your breasts; use firm pressure for the deep tissue in the back. When you've reached the deep tissue, you should be able to feel down to your ribcage. If you have any concerns at all, do not hesitate to visit your family doctor.

Ovarian screening

Currently, in the UK, ovarian cancer screening is not routinely available on the NHS. The reason for this is because evidence suggests that annual surveillance is ineffective in detecting tumours at a sufficiently early stage to reduce the risk of dying from ovarian cancer.[15] However, in some circumstances, particularly in young BRCA mutation carriers who are not yet ready for risk-reducing surgery, such screening may become available.

Over the last decade or so, there have been major UK studies interested in determining whether screening tests such as transvaginal ultrasound examinations and CA-125 blood tests would be useful for diagnosing ovarian cancer. These studies will be discussed in more detail shortly but, before doing so, it is important to understand the screening methods that were included in the trials.

Transvaginal ultrasound

An ultrasound scan of the ovaries uses high frequency sound waves rather than X-rays to obtain pictures of the inside of a patient's body. It is thought to be very safe and generally painless. The scan is typically performed by a radiologist, gynaecologist or sonographer and will last approximately 15 minutes.

There are two different ways of performing a scan. The first looks through the wall of the abdomen (similar to the way a baby is scanned in the womb). The second is to insert a thin probe into the vagina.

A specially designed ultrasound probe is used for this procedure. It is covered with a protective sheath and lubricating gel, before being gently inserted into the vagina. The ultrasound probe needs to be moved in different positions in order to visualise the uterus and ovaries clearly. This method of scanning gives a much clearer picture of the ovaries, womb and surrounding structures and should be no more uncomfortable than having a smear test.

Cancer antigen 125 (CA-125) testing

As mentioned earlier, it is possible to have a blood test to look for a protein called CA-125 which is produced by some ovarian cancer cells; a very high level of CA-125 may suggest that a woman has ovarian cancer. It is present in almost 90% of cases of advanced ovarian cancer, but it is only raised in about half the women who have early stage ovarian cancer.[16]

The CA-125 may be elevated in ovarian cancer, uterine cancer and other intra-abdominal cancers (pancreas, stomach, colon, and rectum) and metastases from other sites (e.g. breast). It is important to be aware that elevated CA-125 may also be associated with non-malignant conditions, such as endometriosis, pregnancy, menstruation and benign ovarian tumours. However, currently it is mainly used when ovarian cancer is suspected and for monitoring after treatment. When levels are elevated, serial monitoring (a series of measurements looking for an increase or decrease in CA-125 levels over time) can be helpful, as rapidly rising levels are more likely to be associated with malignancy than high levels, which are static.

As previously mentioned, currently in the UK, there are two major studies evaluating CA-125 as a screening tool, in combination with other tests. These are the UK Collaborative Trial of Ovarian Cancer Screening study (UKCTOCS) and the UK Familial Ovarian Cancer Screening Study (UK FOCSS).

UK Collaborative Trial of Ovarian Cancer Screening (UKCTOCS)

The UKCTOCS trial[17] is the world's biggest ovarian cancer screening trial, organised by the Gynaecological Cancer Research Centre at University College London (UCL) and supported by Cancer Research UK, the Eve Appeal and the Department of Health, UK.

This 14-year study, which took place between 2001 and 2015, involved over 200,000 women. Its objective was to determine whether or not screening tests would be useful for diagnosing ovarian cancer in the general population and if screening could save lives. If the tests worked well enough it could mean that women with ovarian cancer might be diagnosed earlier, and their cancer treated more effectively. Patients were given either: an annual CA-125 blood test or an annual transvaginal ultrasound scan; or no screening test at all (to reflect the current situation in the UK). Crucially, the CA-125 blood tests were analysed using the 'Risk of Ovarian Cancer Algorithm' (ROCA), which analyses how the levels of CA-125 change over time. Rising levels can indicate that a woman without any symptoms has cancer, but stable or falling levels mean there is a very low risk she currently has cancer. Women with abnormal ROCA test results had repeat CA-125 blood tests and if necessary, ultrasound scans also. This approach was called 'multimodal' screening, because it involved blood tests followed where necessary by ultrasound scans.

The initial results showed that both screening methods ('multimodal' and annual scans) were useful at detecting ovarian cancer before it caused symptoms, but the multimodal screening was superior; there were fewer 'false-positive' screens compared with the annual scans (i.e. fewer women had surgery to remove what turned out to be a benign ovarian tumour rather than cancer). In addition, the ROCA test helped to detect ovarian cancer at earlier stages than the annual scans did.

The trial team continued to follow up these women until 2015 to determine whether or not screening could actually save lives. In December 2015, the much-awaited initial mortality results were released. It was reported that an annual CA-125 blood test might cut ovarian cancer deaths by a fifth.[17] The findings suggested that in patients who were screened by having their CA-125 levels measured every year, and interpreted using the ROCA, ovarian cancer could be detected earlier, giving women a better chance of long-term survival. However, after long-term follow-up to assess the full impact of the screening on women's survival it was reported in 2021 that despite detecting significantly more ovarian cancer at an earlier stage, this did not translate into lives saved.[18] Given that screening did not significantly reduce ovarian and tubal cancer deaths, general population screening cannot be recommended.

UK Familial Ovarian Cancer Screening Study (UK FOCSS)

The UK Familial Ovarian Cancer Screening Study (UK FOCSS) is a screening trial, also organised by the Gynaecological Cancer Research Centre at UCL and supported by Cancer Research UK, the Eve Appeal and the Department of Health, UK.[19]

This 10-year study, which took place between 2002 and 2012, involved over 5000 women at increased risk of ovarian cancer, either because they had a strong family history of the disease or because they were carriers of a BRCA gene mutation. The aim of this study was to find out which screening tests are best for women at high risk of ovarian cancer and to determine how often women should be screened.

In Part 1 of the trial, women who had declined surgery to remove their fallopian tubes and ovaries had an ultrasound scan and a CA-125 blood test once a year. The results showed that women who had longer than a year between screening tests were more likely to be diagnosed with a more advanced cancer. More specifically, the cancers diagnosed were beyond stage 1 in more than 80% of the cases when, ideally, the aim of screening is to detect cancer at its earliest stage when it would be at its most curable.

The trial team concluded that screening once a year may not be often enough to detect early stage ovarian cancer in women at high risk of developing the disease. The researchers decided that it might be better to do screening tests more often than once a year and, therefore, set up Part 2 of the trial in 2007. The women in this part of this trial were given CA-125 tests three times a year (also interpreted using the ROCA as in UKCTOCS) and a transvaginal ultrasound once a year, to determine how effective these tests were.

In February 2017, the results of Part 2 of the trial were released and suggest that screening women at high risk of ovarian cancer every four months may reduce the likelihood of being diagnosed with advanced stage ovarian cancer.[20] During the screening phase of the trial and in the year following their last test, 19 women were diagnosed with ovarian cancer although none had any symptoms. This screening was estimated to have detected more than nine out of 10 cancers before symptoms were apparent. During the follow-up period, in which women were no longer being screened, a further 18 women were diagnosed with ovarian cancer. Seventeen of these 18 women had advanced stage cancer compared with seven of the 19 diagnosed during the screening phase. The results from this study clearly demonstrate that women on the screening programme were significantly less likely to be diagnosed with the most advanced stages of ovarian cancer compared with those who were no longer being screened on the programme.

This study concluded that ROCA-based screening is an option for women at high risk of ovarian and fallopian tube cancer who defer or decline risk-reducing salpingo-oophorectomy. However, it remains unknown whether detecting ovarian cancer by screening increases the chances of a woman surviving the disease.[21] Therefore, women at high risk should still be advised that the safest option is to have risk-reducing surgery. Unlike screening, this is the only intervention which dramatically reduces the risk of developing ovarian cancer.

In response to these results, Athena Lamnisos, Chief Executive of the Eve Appeal, said: 'Knowing that you are at high risk of developing ovarian cancer is a huge stress for women and their families. This research gives women hope and confidence that there is an evidence-based approach to screening if they decide to delay risk-reducing surgery.'[20]

Similar studies have been conducted in the USA and the results of these are likely to be analysed in combination with the results of UKCTOCS and UK FOCSS to inform decisions about whether screening should be offered to high risk women who defer or decline risk-reducing surgery.

Prostate cancer screening

Men who know they carry a BRCA gene mutation can take pro-active steps for some of the cancers associated with the mutation, such as annual prostate cancer screening and annual skin examinations for melanoma. Prostate cancer screening relies on digital rectal examination (DRE) and prostate-specific antigen (PSA) testing.

Digital rectal examination (DRE)

A DRE is a type of physical examination during which a doctor or nurse inserts a finger into the rectum (back passage) to feel for abnormalities of the prostate. If the prostate feels larger than expected for the patient's age, this could be a sign of an enlarged prostate, whereas a prostate with hard bumpy areas might suggest prostate cancer.

PSA testing

Since its introduction in the mid-1980s, the prostate-specific antigen (PSA) test has become a common method of prostate cancer detection. However, because the PSA test is not specific to prostate cancer, and PSA levels can be raised above normal levels in patients with benign conditions, such as infection, its use has caused a lot of controversy.

PSA is a protein produced by both normal and cancerous prostate cells. To check for prostate-specific antigen doctors take a blood sample and may want to rule out urine infection prior to carrying out the test. If there has been a urine infection, a PSA test shouldn't be carried out for at least a month after treatment finishes.

PSA is usually measured in nanograms per millilitre of blood (ng/ml). There is no one PSA reading that is considered normal. The reading varies from man to man and the normal level increases with age; the following values are a rough guide:

- 3 ng/ml or less is considered to be in the normal range for a man under 60 years old;
- 4 ng/ml or less is normal for a man aged 60 to 69;
- 5 ng/ml or less is normal for a man aged over 70.

A reading higher than these values but less than 10 ng/ml is often due to a non-cancerous (benign) enlargement of the prostate gland. A reading higher than 10 ng/ml may also be caused by benign prostate disease, but the higher the level of PSA, the more likely it is to be cancer. However, sometimes a cancer may be diagnosed in a man with a PSA reading within the normal range. Some men have PSA levels in the hundreds (or even thousands) when they are diagnosed with prostate cancer and the higher the level of PSA at diagnosis, the more likely it is the cancer will have spread.

PSA blood tests are also used to decide whether a patient needs treatment and to monitor how well prostate cancer treatment is working. A stable PSA indicates that a cancer is not growing or spreading. If treatment for prostate cancer is successful, the cancer shrinks and, therefore, the PSA level in the blood falls.

With regard to the effectiveness of prostate screening, a review of clinical trials, published in 2010, suggests that routine screening in the general population with either a DRE or PSA does not improve overall survival,[22] but it may help to detect early-stage prostate cancers.

However, with regard to BRCA mutation carriers, initial findings from an ongoing international clinical trial called the IMPACT study, suggests that since male BRCA2 mutation carriers clearly have a much higher risk of early-onset, aggressive prostate cancer, they should be recommended to have PSA testing from the age of 40.[23] However, currently, neither the British nor American urological guidelines recommend that BRCA mutation carriers should be offered such screening. BRCA carriers should speak to their genetics centre and family doctor to determine what is available in their area.

14.
Chemoprevention

Chemoprevention is the use of drugs to prevent or delay the development of cancer. It can be referred to as a prophylactic (preventative) medication.

In June 2013, the National Institute for Health and Care Excellence (NICE) in the UK issued an updated set of clinical guidelines with regard to breast cancer care and treatment, becoming the first European body to recommend that 'at risk' women take preventative drugs for five years in order to decrease their chances of being diagnosed with the condition. They announced that two medications, tamoxifen and raloxifene, would be available on the NHS for women who have a moderate or high risk of developing breast cancer. Women with a family history of breast cancer can now opt to receive a daily dose of tamoxifen or raloxifene which they must take for five years in order to cut the risk of developing breast cancer by half.

However, these medicines do not reduce the risk of hormone-receptor-negative breast cancer – that is, breast cancer that hasn't grown in response to the hormones oestrogen or progesterone.

The NICE decision to recommend that 'at risk' women take preventive drugs is considered a historic one, as previously, women with familial links to breast cancer only had the option of undergoing mastectomy, which can often be an invasive and traumatic experience. Around 488,000 women across the

UK were affected by the new guidelines and the announce-ment gave women more options in terms of managing their increased risk of cancer. Whilst this may be reassuring news to the 3% of women over 35 in the UK eligible for chemopreventive treatment, tamoxifen and raloxifene are not licensed in the UK as preventative treatment for breast cancer. Conversely, the US Food and Drug Administration (FDA) has approved tamoxifen and raloxifene to reduce the risk of breast cancer in women at increased risk.

Both tamoxifen and raloxifene can cause side-effects and they can be more serious in patients taking tamoxifen. These side-effects can be extremely difficult to tolerate, causing many people to stop the drug long before the five years are up. However, some do not experience any side-effects and are able to continue treatment for the recommended period.

Chemoprevention can be discussed and offered to BRCA2 carriers, but should not be offered to BRCA1 carriers due to the potential increased risk of ER-negative breast cancer. Healthcare professionals within a specialist genetic clinic should explain to BRCA2 mutation carriers the possible benefits and harm of taking these drugs so that they can decide whether or not this is an option that they would like to pursue. Discussion and infor-mation should include the side-effects of drugs, the extent of risk reduction, and the risks and benefits of alternative approaches, such as risk-reducing surgery and surveillance. Furthermore, women who've already had mastectomies to remove both breasts won't be offered this chemoprevention because their risk of developing breast cancer is considered to be very low.

Tamoxifen

Tamoxifen fights breast cancer by blocking the action of the hor-mone oestrogen which fuels the growth of some breast cancers. Tamoxifen is probably the most widely used endocrine treatment for breast cancer worldwide, but it is only effective in women with ER-positive (ER+) breast cancer.

Tamoxifen has a molecular shape that is similar to the hormone oestrogen. Some breast tumours contain a molecule that binds oestrogen, called the 'oestrogen receptor' (ER) and when oestrogen binds to the ER molecule it can fuel that cancer's growth. When tamoxifen is used to treat these existing tumours, it appears to block oestrogen from binding to the ER molecule, thereby preventing oestrogen from stimulating further growth.

According to the NICE guideline on familial breast cancer, premenopausal women at high risk of developing breast cancer will be offered tamoxifen for five years unless they have a past history or may be at increased risk of blood clots or endometrial cancer.

Tamoxifen can be combined with oophorectomy for even greater reduction of breast cancer risk, particularly in women with BRCA2 mutations. Evidence suggests that tamoxifen may reduce breast cancer incidence among healthy BRCA2 carriers by 62%, including the risk of cancer in the opposite breast among women previously diagnosed with breast cancer. In contrast, tamoxifen use beginning at age 35 years or older has been found not to reduce breast cancer incidence among healthy women with inherited BRCA1 mutations.[24] While some question the effectiveness in primary prevention in breast cancer in women with BRCA1 mutations, evidence suggests that tamoxifen use is associated with a reduction in contralateral breast cancer risk for both BRCA1 and BRCA2 mutation carriers. That is, tamoxifen is effective in preventing cancer occurring in the second breast after diagnosis of breast cancer in the first breast for both BRCA1 and BRCA2 mutation carriers.[25] Research has recently confirmed that tamoxifen (and raloxifene) reduce the risk of breast cancer coming back (recurrence) during the standard five years of treatment, and that recurrence risk stays lower during the next five years after tamoxifen treatment ends.

While evidence suggests that tamoxifen is very effective in lowering breast cancer risk, its use has been associated with endometrial cancer,[26] blood clots and cataracts, along with quality of life issues like hot flushes which result in many women discontinuing its use long before the five years are up.

Tamoxifen has also been found to cause increased loss of bone mineral density in breast cancer sufferers; however, a differential effect is seen between pre- and postmenopausal women. In premenopausal women with high levels of circulating oestrogen from the ovaries, tamoxifen has an anti-oestrogenic effect which causes increased loss of bone mineral density for one to two years. However, this loss is only about 1-2% and does not continue throughout the five years of tamoxifen therapy. No special monitoring or treatment to prevent this loss is required. In postmenopausal women, on the other hand, tamoxifen has been shown to increase bone mineral density of the spine and hip, but does not increase bone mineral density in the forearm or total body. In summary, the bone loss caused by tamoxifen in premenopausal women does not present a clinical problem requiring bone protecting medication, and tamoxifen protects against bone loss in postmenopausal women.[27]

Raloxifene

Raloxifene is a medicine which is used mostly to prevent and treat osteoporosis in women after the menopause. It is also used to reduce the risk of invasive breast cancer in postmenopausal women with osteoporosis and in postmenopausal women at high risk of invasive breast cancer.

In the UK, raloxifene is currently only licensed for treatment of osteoporosis and is more expensive than tamoxifen, but still constitutes a cost-effective option for the NHS, especially when considering the costs of treating breast cancer.

According to the NICE guidelines, raloxifene may be prescribed for five years to postmenopausal women with a uterus if they have no history or increased risk of blood clots and if they do not wish to take tamoxifen.

Raloxifene has a similar mode of action to tamoxifen, but is being offered as an alternative that may be more helpful to older, post-menopausal women. Raloxifene can cause side-effects including 'flu-like symptoms, hot flushes and leg cramps. Raloxifene has fewer side-effects than tamoxifen, but studies have not examined the effectiveness of raloxifene in preventing breast cancer in BRCA1/2 mutation carriers specifically. However, as previously mentioned, research has recently confirmed that raloxifene reduces the risk of breast cancer coming back during the standard five years of treatment, and that recurrence risk remains lower during the next five years after treatment ends.

Aromatase inhibitors

A class of medicines called aromatase inhibitors are medications that prevent oestrogen production in the adrenal glands, adipose (fat) tissue and brain and may, therefore, help to lower a woman's risk of developing breast cancer. They have fewer side-effects than tamoxifen, but do not work in premenopausal women because they do not prevent the ovaries from producing oestrogen. Examples of aromatase inhibitors include anastrozole (Arimidex), exemestane (Aromasin) and letrozole (Femara).

According to the NICE guidelines, postmenopausal women at high risk of breast cancer will be offered anastrozole for five years unless they have severe osteoporosis.

Oral contraceptives (birth control pills)

Women who take the oral contraceptive pill may benefit from a reduced risk of developing ovarian cancer. This is because the contraceptive pill reduces, or stops completely, the process of ovulation and the fewer the number of menstrual cycles a woman has in her lifetime, the lower her risk of ovarian cancer. Each time a woman ovulates, her ovaries are damaged by the egg as it breaks through the surface of the ovary and is released into her reproductive system. The cells that make up the surface of the ovaries divide and multiply rapidly to repair the damage caused by the egg. It's this rapid cell growth that can occasionally go wrong and result in ovarian cancer. Medications, such as oral contraceptives which stop the process of ovulation can, therefore, help to lessen the chances of developing ovarian cancer.

As in the general population, oral contraceptives have been shown to have a protective effect against ovarian cancer in women with BRCA1/2 mutations.[28] Two large studies have reported risk reductions in the range 38 to 60%, with the maximum observed protection after six or more years of use.[29, 30] In the light of this research, these drugs could be a viable risk-reduction strategy for women who have not completed childbearing or who wish to avoid surgery. However, as with the general population, oral contraceptives have been shown to slightly increase the risk for breast cancer in BRCA mutation carriers.[31] Since women with BRCA mutations are already at high risk of breast cancer, some may be reluctant to take oral contraceptives for fear of increasing their risk of breast cancer.

Women considering taking oral contraceptives should discuss the risks and benefits with their doctor.

15.
Risk-reducing surgery

Risk-reducing surgery involves removing healthy tissue which is at high risk of developing cancer. For those women who choose to undergo risk-reducing surgery in the management of their BRCA mutation, the options available include surgical removal of their breast tissue, known as a mastectomy, and surgical removal of their ovaries and fallopian tubes, known as a salpingo-oophorectomy. In this respect, risk-reducing surgery involves removing as much of the 'at risk' tissue as possible, hopefully before any cancer has developed.

Female BRCA mutation carriers who are at high risk of developing breast and ovarian cancer are often faced with the difficult decision of whether or not to remove these tissues. Deciding if and when to have risk-reducing surgeries is an intensely personal decision and it is important for women to consult with experts in genetics, gynaecologic oncology and breast surgery. These specialists will help you to make the best decision that is right for you in managing your risk of cancer.

It is important to remember that risk-reducing surgery does not completely guarantee that cancer will not develop because not all of the at-risk tissue can be removed by these surgeries. Some women have developed breast, ovarian, or primary peritoneal cancer (a type of cancer similar to ovarian cancer) even after this type of surgery. Nevertheless, the reduction in cancer mortality associated with having undergone these surgeries is substantial. For example, a study published in 2010 found that women who underwent bilateral salpingo-oophorectomy had a nearly 80% reduction in risk of dying from ovarian cancer and more than a 50% reduction in risk of dying from breast cancer.[32]

Bilateral salpingo-oophorectomy (BSO)

The surgical procedure to remove both the fallopian tubes and ovaries is known as a bilateral salpingo-oophorectomy (BSO) and may also be referred to as a risk-reducing salpingo-oophorectomy (RRSO). Almost 4000 women in the UK undergo this surgery each year.[33]

A BSO is typically performed laparoscopically using two or three small incisions, or by open surgery using one large incision. During laparoscopic surgery, the surgeon makes a very small cut (incision), usually in the belly button, and two other small incisions will be made on the lower abdomen. A tube is inserted through the incision in the belly button and carbon dioxide gas is pumped through the tube to inflate the abdomen; this allows the surgeon to see the organs more clearly and gives them more room to work. The surgeon then inserts a tiny camera, known as a laparoscope, through this tube. The camera transmits video to a television monitor that the surgeon watches so that s/he can guide the surgical tools. Small, surgical instruments can then be inserted through the other two incisions and the surgeon can guide them to the right place using the view from the laparoscope. Each ovary can then be separated from the blood supply and surrounding tissue and removed through one of the incisions. In some cases, surgery that begins as laparoscopic may end up as an open procedure if the surgeon deems it necessary. Furthermore, open procedures are usually used in women with a high BMI or previous abdominal surgery which can cause adhesions (internal scar tissue which can result in bodily tissues sticking together) to form internally, making keyhole surgery very difficult.

Due to the limitations of screening for ovarian cancer, women at increased risk often consider risk-reducing surgery. BSO is the single most effective method for reducing the risk of ovarian cancer and for reducing mortality from ovarian cancer in BRCA mutation carriers. It has been shown to reduce ovarian cancer risk in BRCA mutation carriers by up to 96%.[34] Furthermore, evidence suggests that women with BRCA mutations who undergo removal of their ovaries before the natural menopause may also benefit from up to a 50% breast cancer risk reduction.[35] This is because removing the ovaries takes away the body's main source of the hormone oestrogen, which is known to fuel the growth of some breast cancers. In addition to this, removing the ovaries also significantly decreases a woman's production of testosterone, an important hormone for health, wellbeing and libido. However, removing the ovaries will not affect production of testosterone in the adrenal glands.

It is advised that women with BRCA mutations be referred to a gynaecologic oncologist to discuss the option of BSO and, ideally, initial consultation should take place when the woman approaches her mid-30s. Women are recommended to undergo BSO preferably between 35 and 40 years or upon completion of childbearing because the incidence of ovarian cancer rises sharply after this age. However, if there is a familial history of BRCA-related cancers occurring at a particularly young age, it may be advisable to consider risk-reducing surgery earlier. Currently in the UK, women with BRCA mutations who decide to undergo risk-reducing surgery are typically advised to do so no later than five to 10 years before the youngest age of breast and/or ovarian cancer in the family, so long as childbearing is complete.

After undergoing a BSO, a woman will experience a surgical-ly-induced menopause and will be sterile. She will, therefore, be unable to bear a child. However, infertility services can be used to preserve a woman's eggs but, given that the benefits of the surgery are greatest close to menopause, most women simply postpone the surgery until they have already borne as many children as they wish.

While BSO lowers the risk of ovarian cancer, it does not entirely eliminate it. Firstly, this is because some women who are at high risk may already have ovarian cancer at the time of risk-reducing surgery. The cancer can be so small that it is only found when the ovaries are viewed under a microscope. Secondly, in some women with endometriosis, it can prove very difficult to detach and remove the ovary and fallopian tubes intact from the surrounding organs. This is because endometriosis makes the tissue which normally grows inside the uterus grow outside it, causing the uterus, ovaries and fallopian tubes to stick together. As a result, pieces of the ovary or fallopian tubes may be unavoidably left behind after surgery and may be at risk of developing malignancy. Furthermore, even after ovary removal, there is a small chance that patients could go on to develop primary peritoneal cancer (page 82) which is indistinguishable from ovarian cancer. This is because, as previously mentioned, the lining of the abdomen and the surface of the ovary come from the same tissue when we develop from embryos in the womb.

In addition to undergoing a BSO, high-risk women often face the very difficult decision of whether also to have their uterus removed. While the current recommendation in the UK for BRCA mutation carriers is to leave the uterus intact, some may choose to have a BSO in conjunction with a hysterectomy to remove the uterus. This is especially true for women who want to take tamoxifen to lower their risk for breast cancer because this drug is known to cause uterine cancer. Furthermore, since there is an increased risk of fallopian tube cancer in BRCA mutation carriers and because a remnant of the fallopian tube is left in the uterine wall at the time of BSO, there is a theoretical benefit in considering a total abdominal hysterectomy as this remnant of tube will then also be removed along with the uterus. However, hysterectomy would carry with it additional risks and recovery time compared with a BSO alone.[36]

Despite BSO being the most effective way of lowering the risk of ovarian cancer, evidence suggests that many women are unwilling to undergo such risk-reducing surgery. A study which investigated uptake of RRSO in 700 BRCA mutation carriers from Greater Manchester, England, found that uptake in BRCA1 mutation carriers was 54.5% at five years post-testing, compared with 45.5% for BRCA2 mutation carriers. The greatest uptake was in the 40–59 year-old category, but uptake was significantly lower in the over 60s which, researchers say, may be due to the perception that if they have not developed cancer yet they will not develop it in the future. However, because there is no efficient method for early detection of ovarian cancer, researchers suggest that, ideally, uptake should be greater.[37] In contrast, in the US, as many as 70% of women who learn they have BRCA mutations choose to undergo risk-reducing oophorectomy.[38]

Early risk-reducing salpingectomy and delayed oophorectomy – an alternative risk-reducing strategy?

As mentioned on page 76, originally, all ovarian cancers were believed to develop in the lining of the ovary as a result of the constant rupture and repair process during ovulation. However, some doctors now think that most ovarian cancers typically seen in BRCA mutation carriers may actually start in the part of the tube closest to the ovary (the distal end of the tube).

Based on this, an alternative risk-reducing strategy has been put forward: early risk-reducing salpingectomy and delayed oophorectomy. Some experts have proposed that 'interval salpingectomy' – removing the fallopian tubes and leaving the ovaries intact until after natural menopause – might lower the risk for ovarian cancer in high-risk women. This would avoid the negative side-effects and long-term health consequences associated with oophorectomy at a young age, such as the increased risk of osteoporosis and heart disease, among others.[39, 40]

However, the efficacy and safety of this alternative strategy need further investigation. Given that 15-30% of serous ovarian cancers show no evidence of fallopian tube involvement (suggesting that the cancer may have originated on the ovarian surface), interval salpingectomy would offer little prospect of risk-reduction against cancers which develop in this way.[41] Furthermore, a second surgery to remove the ovaries presents additional risks and there is a concern about whether interval salpingectomy might provide BRCA mutation carriers with a false sense of security about their risk of cancer, leading to a significant delay or even a rejection of definitive oophorectomy.

However, currently in the UK, the standard of treatment still remains salpingo-oophorectomy between the ages of 35 and 40, or after childbearing is complete, as it is this strategy which offers the greatest reduction in risk for breast and ovarian cancer among BRCA mutation carriers.[42]

Finally, for those women who are not currently prepared to have their ovaries removed, such as for those whose families are not yet complete, there are a number of other possibilities which should be discussed with a gynaecologist. For example, depending on a woman's specific circumstances, a gynaecologist might consider the removal of a single fallopian tube or the possibility of ovum (egg) freezing, a procedure in which a woman's eggs can be retrieved and then frozen with the goal of being used in the future when the patient is ready to start a family. In all cases, advice should be sought from a gynaecologist and genetic counsellor to discuss these less common options.

Surgically induced menopause

The menopause is sometimes referred to as 'the change of life' and is the name given to the end of menstruation (periods). This can happen naturally, or it can be surgically induced.

Women who have their ovaries removed, and who are not yet menopausal, will experience a surgically induced menopause and premature oestrogen deficiency. Early menopause is associated with short-term and long-term symptoms, both of which may potentially affect a woman's quality of life. Symptoms of the menopause, according to the NHS,[43] may include:

- hot flushes and night sweats;
- difficulty sleeping;
- mood changes, such as low mood or anxiety;
- headaches;
- vaginal dryness;
- reduced sex drive (libido);
- urinary tract infection;
- sexual difficulties;
- weight gain;
- joint stiffness, aches and pains;
- dry skin;
- hair loss;
- reduced energy and fitness;
- difficulty with word recall.

These symptoms, caused by a lack of oestrogen in the body, may be mild or severe and there is no way of predicting their severity. However, most of these symptoms can be treated, at least partially, with many women taking HRT. Often, after BSO, younger women may safely take HRT to manage menopausal symptoms and derive other oestrogen-related benefits through to the age that natural menopause would have taken place, which, on average, is around the age of 51 years.

However, not all of these symptoms are directly related to the menopause. Some are part of the natural ageing process and are experienced by both men and women.

Hormone replacement therapy (HRT)
When a woman's ovaries are removed, her levels of oestrogen and progesterone will drop significantly. This may negatively affect her health and quality of life. HRT replaces those hormones which would have normally been produced by the ovaries, albeit to a lower level than normal.

Women with premature menopause are commonly prescribed HRT, and are advised to continue taking it until at least age 50. Women who keep their uterus intact at the time of BSO may be given combined therapy of oestrogen and progesterone because oestrogen given alone increases the risk of uterine cancer. Giving progesterone and oestrogen in combination seems to counteract the adverse effect of oestrogen and helps to protect the health of the uterus. However, women who choose to have their uterus removed at the time of BSO may be given oestrogen-only HRT (known as 'unopposed oestrogen' as the oestrogen is not modified by the effects of progesterone).

HRT is available in tablet, skin patch, gel or six-month implant form. In some women, it may be a case of trial and error before finding the form of HRT that is best suited to them. There has been a lot written about HRT, its side-effects and links to other diseases – however, it can be effective in treating several of the most common menopausal symptoms.

HRT generally reduces hot flushes, night sweats and vaginal dryness related to surgical menopause and improves sexual functioning. However, in some women, particularly young women, vaginal dryness may continue to be a problem even during HRT. Vaginal dryness is a direct result of lowered oestrogen levels, but women who experience it may find that low-dose oestrogen creams, low-dose tablets, or an oestrogen-releasing device called a 'low-dose vaginal oestrogen ring' to be helpful. These work by delivering oestrogen to the vaginal walls, reversing changes due to lack of hormones and helping to improve lubrication while minimising absorption into the body.

HRT can also help prevent osteoporosis and in young women it may reduce the risk of cardiovascular disease. Although evidence suggests that bilateral oophorectomy before the age of 50 doubles the risk of developing cardiovascular disease,[44] the use of HRT appears to eliminate this increased risk. Evidence also suggests that oophorectomy increases the risk of osteoporotic fracture by 50%, but HRT was also found to reduce the risk of fracture.[45]

Reassuringly, a study published in 2014 which looked at hormone therapy in BRCA1 and BRCA2 mutation carriers who had undergone oophorectomy found that short-term HRT improved their quality of life and did not seem to have an adverse effect on cancer risk in those who had no personal history of breast cancer.[46] However, for women who do not wish to take HRT, or who cannot for medical reasons, there are other treatments which may ease the symptoms of the menopause and promote good health for the future. Such women should seek advice from their family doctor, gynaecologist or menopause specialist.

Osteoporosis

Osteoporosis, which literally means 'porous bones', is a medical condition in which the bones become brittle and fragile. This typically occurs as a result of hormonal changes or dietary deficiencies in calcium, vitamin D or magnesium. Osteoporosis currently affects one in every three women in Western society.[47] Risk factors associated with the development of osteoporosis include a family history of the disease, being underweight or of small and thin stature, smoking, excessive alcohol, early menopause and the use of certain medications, such as steroids.

It is often called the silent epidemic as many people are unaware of its onset and the first indication of the disease can be falling and breaking a bone. In general, people with a bone mineral density significantly lower than that normal for their age and gender are more likely to break a bone, even with very minor trauma such as falling from a small height or violent sneezing and coughing.

Bones continue to grow and develop throughout childhood and adolescence and the bones are at their most dense around the age of 30 but, beyond this age, bone mass gradually diminishes. Osteoporosis is considered a natural part of ageing although with treatment it is largely preventable. Osteoporosis can affect people of both sexes and all ages, although older, post-menopausal women are particularly at risk. This is because after the menopause the level of oestrogen declines, resulting in a decrease in bone density. Osteoporosis is estimated to be six to eight times more common in women than in men as women have a lower bone mass to start with.[47] Because of this, bone mass density testing is recommended for all women over the age of 65.

Women who have undergone surgery to remove their ovaries but do not take HRT may be at increased risk of developing osteoporosis. In the UK, women who are considering oophorectomy are recommended to have a baseline bone mineral density test before they undergo surgery to determine how strong their bones are to begin with. The findings from this scan can then be compared with future scans, after their ovaries have been removed, to identify any loss in bone density. However, in the UK there are no hard and fast rules as to the recommended frequency of subsequent bone density scans, but factors such as HRT use, bone density at baseline and patient's age will influence the recommended frequency of such screening.

A bone density scan, such as a DEXA scan, is a special type of X-ray that measures the calcium content of the bone. The examination is usually performed on the lower spine and the hips. It is a simple, quick and non-invasive medical test, which involves exposing particular parts of the body to very small amounts of radiation. Doctors use the results to help them decide whether treatment for low bone density is needed. If evidence of osteopenia (a condition in which bone density is lower than normal, considered by many doctors to be a precursor to osteoporosis) or osteoporosis exists, then bisphosphonate treatment may need to be started. This helps to maintain or increase bone density and strength, thereby preventing the development of osteoporosis.

There are various lifestyle choices that can help improve bone health, such as exercise and diet. Exercise is recommended as this helps to strengthen bones. However, the type of exercise is very important; it should be regular and it should be weight bearing. This is because weight-bearing exercise encourages the loading of calcium into the bones, helping to keep them strong and healthy. This includes any type of exercise that involves upright movement so that pressure is exerted through the spine, pelvis and legs. Walking, jogging, aerobics, yoga, dancing and climbing stairs are all examples of weight-bearing exercise. On the other hand, swimming and cycling are not. Although these activities help build and maintain strong muscles and have excellent cardiovascular benefits, they are not the best form of exercise to help maintain strong bones.

Diet is also particularly important; it should contain high levels of calcium, vitamin D and magnesium. High calcium foods include dark leafy greens (for example, curly kale, spinach and broccoli), cheese, low fat milk and yogurt, okra, green beans, almonds, and fish canned with their bones. Vitamin D is an essential vitamin required by the body for the absorption of calcium. Natural foods high in vitamin D include oily fish (salmon, mackerel), mushrooms, cheese, and egg yolks. In addition, vitamin D is widely added to many foods such as milk, cereals and orange juice. Vitamin D is also naturally made by the body when the skin is exposed to the sun. Exposing only a forearm length of skin to the sun's ultraviolet rays for around 20 minutes each day will produce adequate vitamin D to help maintain bone density. However, for those who spend a lot of time indoors, it may be necessary to take a vitamin D supplement. Furthermore, what is less well known is that magnesium also plays an important part in maintaining bone density as it is needed to aid the absorption of calcium. Natural foods high in magnesium include spinach, almonds, avocado and dark chocolate.

However, before starting any exercise regimen or making any dietary changes, please seek medical advice from a doctor.

Sexual dysfunction

After risk-reducing salpingo-oophorectomy, some women may develop sexual difficulties. A study published in 2016 which aimed to determine the prevalence of sexual dysfunction in women after BSO and to assess factors which may influence sexual wellbeing following this surgery, reported that the prevalence of female sexual dysfunction (FSD) was 74% and the prevalence of hypoactive sexual desire disorder (HSDD) – a lack of sexual fantasies and desire for sexual activity – was 73%. Common sexual issues experienced included:

- lubrication difficulty (44%);
- reduced sexual satisfaction (41%);
- pain during sexual intercourse (dyspareunia) (28%);
- orgasm difficulty (25%).

However, factors such as relationship satisfaction and the use of topical vaginal oestrogen were significantly associated with a decreased likelihood of sexual dysfunction.[48]

While it is alarming that evidence suggests the risk of sexual dysfunction is high after ovary removal, not all women who undergo this surgery experience it. But, in those that do, there are various strategies which can be employed to help resolve the problem, including specialist counselling, the use of HRT (if appropriate) and vaginal oestrogen creams to improve lubrication. Furthermore, women who experience a loss of libido, and who do not respond to HRT, may, in some cases, be prescribed testosterone by their gynaecologist, in the hope that it will boost libido.[49]

Reassuringly, evidence suggests that many of the adverse effects experienced by women after removal of the ovaries improve significantly between six and 12 months after surgery, with many returning to normal functioning within one year.[50]

Any women struggling with sexual dysfunction after risk-reducing surgery should not suffer unnecessarily and should seek advice from their family doctor or the relevant specialists.

Weight gain

As oestrogen levels drop during menopause, the metabolism slows down. As a result, the body burns fewer calories and stores more fat. With this in mind, only naturally many women facing the difficult decision of having their ovaries removed will worry about weight gain.

However, while weight gain may occur with the menopause, younger women who become menopausal do not tend to experience it in the same way as older patients do. The possibility of weight gain tends to be an age-related issue that is related to lifestyle factors, such as a poor diet or a lack of exercise. Eating a healthy diet which is high in fibre, low in saturated fats, limiting the intake of alcohol and participating in regular exercise will help towards maintaining a healthy body weight. Furthermore, women who take an adequate dose of HRT will not experience changes to their metabolism, which will remain the same as when their ovaries were intact.

Reassuringly, a study published in 2015 of 1454 BRCA mutation carriers which compared the bodyweight of women with and without oophorectomy, found that there was only a small and non-significant difference between those who had had an oophorectomy and those who had not; it concluded, therefore, that oophorectomy is not associated with significant weight gain.[51]

Quality of life

Aside from the potential medical benefits of BSO, very little is known about women's quality of life following surgery.

Women who undergo BSO have reported various physical and psychological consequences, including post-operative complications, the onset of menopausal symptoms, side-effects of HRT, and negative effects on body image and sexuality (capacity for sexual feelings).[52] On the other hand, evidence also suggests that, for women who do not undergo a BSO, continued screening at regular intervals, with the ongoing worry over the possibility of detecting an abnormality each time, increases anxiety which, in turn, decreases quality of life.[53]

Reassuringly, however, evidence suggests that overall quality of life in women following BSO is comparable to that of the general population. A study published in 2009 aimed to investigate quality of life and fatigue in 450 women who had undergone risk-reducing salpingo-oophorectomy. Women were asked to complete a questionnaire which contained measures of quality of life, fatigue, anxiety/depression, body image and morbidity (incidence of disease), among others. Researchers found that women who had undergone BSO showed similar levels of quality of life and fatigue as those of the same age who had not undergone BSO. However, women who had had cancer before BSO had lower levels of quality of life and more fatigue than women without cancer.[54] Similarly, the study found that women who had undergone BSO had lower levels of depression and total mental distress compared with individuals in the general population. However, women who had undergone BSO had more palpitations, constipation, pain and stiffness, osteoporosis and musculoskeletal disease than the general population, even after taking into account the use of HRT.[54] Another study published in the same year, which aimed to compare quality of life in women who had undergone RRSO with those who had had screening, found that although women in the surgery group were more likely to report hot flushes and vaginal dryness, most of the reported adverse effects were no longer apparent within six to 12 months after surgery. Furthermore, no differences in body image or depressive symptoms were observed between the two groups at any point.[50]

Cognitive impairment

Cognitive impairment refers to a noticeable and measurable decline in cognitive abilities, including memory and thinking skills. Most healthy people experience a gradual decline in mental abilities as part of ageing. However, scientists have found a link between cognitive impairment and oophorectomy. Research led by Dr Gilliam Einstein monitored 133 women between the ages of 35 and 50, measuring their cognitive ability with a series of tests for at least three years. One third of the women had surgery to remove both of their ovaries, another third carried the BRCA-gene mutation but did not undergo the operation and the final third were healthy volunteers. The study found that those who had had their ovaries removed performed worse in word-recall tests and logical memory tests, with some showing a growing decline for eight years after the surgery. This decline was not seen in the other two groups. However, women who had been given HRT showed less evidence of decline.[55] Oestrogen, according to Dr Einstein, is crucial in securing brain health in women. Katherine Taylor, chief executive at Ovarian Cancer Action, told *MailOnline*: 'We welcome research that builds on our knowledge of BRCA and cancer prevention but urge women with BRCA gene mutations not to panic in the light of this new research, which is in its early stages. If you're offered ovarian removal surgery and face a premature menopause you will usually also be offered HRT.'[55]

Furthermore, in addition to the high risk of developing breast and ovarian cancer, evidence suggests that a BRCA1 gene mutation, in itself, may contribute to neurological disorders, including Alzheimer's disease, the irreversible, progressive brain disorder that slowly destroys memory and thinking skills. In a study, published in 2015, researchers discovered considerably reduced levels of BRCA1 protein in the brains of patients with Alzheimer's disease, suggesting that the BRCA1 gene plays an essential part in keeping brain cells healthy.[56] However, further research is required to determine whether people with a BRCA1 gene mutation are more likely to develop Alzheimer's disease.

Cardiovascular disease

Cardiovascular disease (CVD) is a general term for conditions affecting the heart or blood vessels, including coronary heart disease, angina, heart attack and stroke, among others.

The risk of developing heart disease may increase in menopausal women as there is no oestrogen to protect against hardening of the arteries and other heart problems. Oestrogen is believed to have a positive effect on the inner layer of the artery wall, helping to keep blood vessels flexible, which means that they can relax and expand to accommodate blood flow. Indeed, the use of HRT has been shown to lower the risk of developing heart disease among menopausal women.[57]

Evidence suggests that a lack of oestrogen, resulting from the menopause, is associated with higher risks of cardiovascular disease.[57] However, a more recent study allays fears that oophorectomy may increase the risk of cardiovascular disease. This study used data collected from SWAN, the Study of Women's Health Across the Nation, designed to examine the health of women during their middle years, followed thousands of women before, during and after menopause. More than

3300 women aged 42-52 were enrolled in the study and then followed for about 11 years. Between 1996 and 2008, just over half the women had reached menopause and 183 had undergone a hysterectomy or a hysterectomy plus oophorectomy. After looking at cardiovascular risk factors like cholesterol and blood pressure, researchers found that a hysterectomy with or without oophorectomy was not strongly associated with risk for heart disease. Although further research is needed to establish a better understanding of how these medical procedures may affect heart health, findings to date are promising.[58]

It is important to know that cardiovascular disease is a multi-factorial disease, meaning it results from a number of factors, including both genetic and environmental. Eating a healthy diet rich in fruit and vegetables, regular exercise, being a non-smoker and maintaining a healthy body weight will all help to lower the risk of developing cardiovascular disease. Furthermore, those who have followed a healthy lifestyle, and continue doing so at menopause, will have a lower risk for heart disease and stroke.[59]

Bilateral mastectomy

A 'bilateral mastectomy' is the term for the removal of both breasts by a breast surgeon and may also include removal of the nipple and areola. Risk-reducing mastectomy is recommended for women who have a strong family history of breast cancer or for individuals who test positive for certain genetic mutations, such as those in the BRCA1 and BRCA2 genes.

It is the single most effective way of reducing the risk of developing breast cancer and, in high-risk women, can reduce the risk 90-95%.[2] However, the amount of reduction in risk that is achieved is dependent upon a number of factors. The surgeon has to balance removing as much breast tissue as possible without damaging the delicate blood vessels which supply the overlying skin. There are factors to do with the breast itself that alter how close to the skin the surgeon can dissect; patient factors to do with the health of the patient, and surgeon factors, such as their experience. Therefore, not all risk-reducing mastectomies will be identical but, irrespective of the differences, they will all remove the vast majority of breast tissue.

It is important to remember that while risk-reducing mastectomy is highly effective in reducing the risk of breast cancer, this surgery offers a risk reduction and *not* risk elimination. No matter how thorough the surgeon is, it is not possible to remove every last breast cell and, therefore, there is still a small residual risk of developing cancer in the small amount of tissue that remains.

In the UK, all BRCA mutation carriers will be given the opportunity to discuss risk-reducing mastectomy with an experienced breast surgeon and should be made aware that there are several techniques available for mastectomy and for breast reconstruction following surgery. Furthermore, all carriers are entitled to more than one surgical opinion. Women can also be referred to a psychologist if discussions regarding impact on body image would aid decision-making.

The techniques that are available for risk-reducing mastectomies include:

- **simple mastectomy** removes all of the breast tissue and most of the skin covering the breasts, leaving the least amount of breast tissue in the body; therefore, achieving the greatest risk reduction. It may be recommended for women not having breast reconstruction. In addition to risk-reducing use, it is also used by women who have been diagnosed with earlier stages of cancer;
- **skin-sparing mastectomy** removes all of the breast tissue, including the nipple and areola, but leaves the 'excess' skin in place for reconstruction. It has less visible scar tissue than a simple mastectomy;
- **nipple-sparing mastectomy** is a skin-sparing mastectomy which removes the breast tissue, but leaves the

nipple and areola intact for a more natural appearance. The scars may be hidden in the infra-mammary fold under the breast;

- **areola-sparing mastectomy** removes the breast tissue and the nipple, but not the areola. This mastectomy removes the small amount of ductal tissue within the nipple, whilst leaving a natural-looking areola;
- **nerve-sparing mastectomy** is a procedure which maintains the nerves that provide sensation to the skin over the breasts. Breasts that have undergone any of these surgeries have much less tactile sensation than natural breasts. Nerve-sparing techniques are an effort to retain some feeling in the breasts, with limited and often only partial success.

When performing a mastectomy, the surgeon may use one of the following three types of incision:

1. infra-mammary incision – at the base of the breast, near the chest wall; an inconspicuous scar;
2. transaxillary incision – in the armpit; therefore no scar on the breast;
3. periareolar incision – around the lower side of the areola (the darkened tissue around the nipple); leaving a small and discreet scar.

However, women who decide to undergo breast-size reductions at the time of mastectomy will have longer and different incisions. For example, a surgeon might remove 1000 grams of breast tissue but only reconstruct with a 500 cc implant. Therefore, the skin is reduced during the procedure and rewrapped over the smaller breast. In these women, an 'inverted T' incision may be used and the resulting scar ends up looking like an anchor (or an upside-down letter 'T').

The chosen mastectomy technique is determined by the

existence of any cancer and overall health, as well as by the woman's desire, if any, for breast reconstruction surgery for aesthetic purposes. Women who choose a flat-chested appearance or use external breast prostheses typically choose simple mastectomy, with its greater risk reduction. However, a nipple-sparing risk-reducing mastectomy in which the nipple is not removed is being increasingly performed as an option for women at high risk for breast cancer, and may offer better cosmetic results than a skin-sparing risk-reducing mastectomy where the nipple-areola complex is removed. This type of mastectomy is being increasingly performed via the infra-mammary fold (IMF) – the fold at the base of the breast where the breast and the chest meet – so that any scarring will be hidden in the fold.

However, patients are warned that there may be a residual breast cancer risk due to the maintained nipple-areola complex, although this risk is thought to be low. While a residual cancer risk exists, it is very difficult to quantify and at present there is no solid evidence to clarify this. As a result, it would be important for any woman planning on having a nipple-sparing mastectomy to discuss this residual risk with her surgeon. Nonetheless, a study published in 2015 concluded that a nipple-sparing mastectomy is an acceptable choice for patients with BRCA mutations. It found no evidence of compromise to oncological safety at short-term follow-up of between approximately one and three-and-a-half years after surgery. Furthermore, complication rates were acceptable and subsequent removal of the nipple-areola complex was rarely required.[60]

Decision making

Deciding whether or not to undergo a risk-reducing mastectomy is a major decision and, naturally, women who are facing such surgery will be fearful of the impact this could have on their sexuality, quality of life and feelings of regret subsequently. It is known that mastectomy due to breast cancer is associated with chronic pain and a negative impact on sexuality and this may also be the same experience of women who undergo risk-reducing mastectomy.

A study published in 2015 aimed to determine if sparing the nipple-areola complex during risk-reducing mastectomy would impact on cancer-related distress and body image. They found that women who had undergone nipple-areola-sparing mastectomy had significantly higher levels of satisfaction with breasts and with the outcome generally, and sexual wellbeing compared with those women who had undergone skin-sparing mastectomy. No statistically significant differences in total cancer-related distress, anxiety or depression were observed between the two groups.[61] However, given that a residual risk remains with leaving the nipple-areola complex intact, some women may choose to have their nipple-areola complex removed during mastectomy, in order to reduce their risk of developing breast cancer as much as possible.

Unfortunately, women who undergo mastectomy are likely to experience considerable loss in skin and nipple-areola complex sensation following surgery. A study published in 2016 which aimed to evaluate sensation and patient satisfaction after nipple-sparing or skin-sparing mastectomy found that both groups of patients had significant reduction in skin sensation. For those who underwent a nipple-sparing mastectomy, measurable nipple and areola sensation was preserved in both breasts for 26% of patients and in one breast for 68% of patients. However, neither group reported being satisfied with sexual arousal with breast or nipple stimulation after surgery.[62]

However, a study published in 2000 which aimed to evaluate patients' long-term satisfaction and psychological and social function following risk-reducing mastectomy in over 600 women, reported that most women (70%) were satisfied with the procedure. The most striking finding was that 74% of women had decreased emotional concern about developing breast cancer after risk-reduction surgery. The majority of women reported generally favourable psychological and social outcomes, including no change/favourable effects in levels of emotional stability (68%/23%), stress (58%/28%), self-esteem (69%/13%), sexual relationships (73%/4%) and feelings of femininity (67%/8%). Altogether, 48% reported no change in their level of satisfaction with body appearance; 16% reported favourable effects.[63] Furthermore, a study published in 2008 reported no anxiety or depression and no negative effects on quality of life after surgery, although 48% of women reported feeling less sexually attractive.[64]

Women who undergo mastectomy (or lumpectomy) may experience long-term nerve pain, referred to as post-mastectomy pain syndrome (PMPS). Studies have shown that between 20% and 60% of women develop PMPS after surgery, but it is often not recognised as such. The classic signs of PMPS are chest wall pain and tingling down the arm. Pain may also be felt in the shoulder, scar, arm or armpit. Other common complaints include numbness, shooting or pricking pain, or unbearable itching. PMPS is thought to be linked to damage done to the nerves in the armpit and chest during surgery, but the exact causes are not known.[65] A study published in 2010 aimed to analyse the prevalence of pain and discomfort in the breasts, impact on sexuality, quality of life, and feelings of regret after bilateral risk-reducing mastectomy and immediate reconstruction with implants. The results showed that 69% reported pain and 71% discomfort in the breasts. Lost or much reduced sexual sensations were reported by 85% and enjoyment of sex was negatively affected for 75% of patients. However, quality of life was reportedly not affected and feelings of regret were almost non-existent. In conclusion, researchers noted the importance of informing women approaching this risk-reducing procedure about the risk of having unwanted secondary effects.[66]

Reconstruction after mastectomy

The goal of breast reconstruction is to recreate the shape and form of a breast, thereby helping to give patients the self-esteem and confidence to lead a normal life. Indeed, the most common reason for breast reconstruction is for the patient's psychological wellbeing.

Determining the many variables of breast reconstruction surgery can be daunting and the appropriateness of a certain type of breast reconstruction will depend on a patient's overall health, breast size and shape, and their personal preferences.

Breast reconstruction is usually done by a plastic surgeon, and may be done as part of the same multi-hour surgery that removes the breasts. There are multiple techniques that may be used in breast reconstruction, with different locations and amounts of scarring. However, breast reconstruction has evolved towards less invasive, single-stage procedures.[67]

The two most common forms of breast reconstruction patients receive are:

1. implant-based, using a tissue expander/implant;
2. tissue-flap reconstruction, where your own tissue is used.

There is also the matter of determining whether the patient will undergo immediate or delayed reconstructive surgery.

Implant-based reconstruction

The simplest way of reconstructing the breast is with breast implants. There are two main types of implant available: silicone gel implants and saline implants. They are both made of a rubbery silicone envelope, but one is filled with silicone gel and the other with sterile salt water (saline). Both have a long history of use, but the silicone implant is softer, is less prone to wrinkling and feels more natural.

In breast reconstruction, the implants may be placed either

above the chest muscle (sub-glandular) or beneath it (sub-muscular). However, the majority of plastic surgeons place breast implants below the muscle as the muscle provides additional coverage over the breast implant which is especially important to give a smooth transition in the upper chest/breast area. Also, it will prevent the implant from being visible and help to camouflage rippling and wrinkling of the implant which is especially important in very slim women.

Implant-based reconstruction can either be performed as a single-stage procedure in which the implant is inserted immediately after mastectomy, known as an immediate reconstruction, or as a staged approach to implant reconstruction, known as a delayed-immediate reconstruction. In most women who have undergone a mastectomy the skin overlying the chest wall is too tight to perform an immediate reconstruction. Therefore, the plastic surgeon places a tissue expander, which is a temporary implant that's more like a balloon. It stretches the skin to make room for the final implant and allows a woman to expand her natural breast size to a larger size. The expander has a special port that allows the surgeon to add increasing amounts of salt water solution over time (typically between two and three months) until the skin gradually is stretched enough to accommodate the final implant. When the woman has achieved her desired size, she will then undergo further surgery to remove the tissue expanders and to replace them with silicone implants.

Surgeons who reconstruct using implants are also likely to use 'acellular dermal matrices' (ADMs) which act as an internal 'bra'. An ADM is a biological mesh derived from animal skin which has been processed to make it completely safe to use in humans. It provides an additional layer of tissue between the skin and the implant. The implant will be covered by the patient's own muscle at the top and by the mesh at the bottom. This approach means that a much more natural shape can be achieved in this type of reconstruction. However, while there are clear benefits to their use, they are very costly to the NHS. Given that implants and ADMs may not last a lifetime, patients who undergo implant based reconstruction are likely to require further surgery at some point in the future.

This type of reconstruction would be suitable for those patients who prefer to avoid more invasive, lengthy procedures which have more scarring. The main advantages of implant-based reconstruction are, first, that it is a relatively quick operation (around one and a half hours) which does not subject the patient to too much surgical trauma and, second, patients only tend to be in hospital for one night and have a quicker recovery time of around two weeks, as well as less scarring than other types of reconstruction. The downside is that the breast won't feel as natural as it would if made with living tissue. It is likely to be firmer, less mobile and feel colder.

The main disadvantages of implant-based reconstruction include the possibility of experiencing:

- bottoming out, which occurs when the breast implant drops below the level of the breast causing a bulge in the wrong place, making any infra-mammary scars visible on the breast;
- rippling, or wrinkling in the skin, which is believed to be caused by the breast implant pulling on the scar tissue which develops around it, which pulls on the skin, causing a rippling appearance;
- capsular contracture – a breast implant is a foreign body and, as with all implanted foreign bodies, the immune system responds to it by encasing it in a very thin fibrous layer. Often, this capsule will be of no consequence but, in some patients, and for reasons unknown, the fibrous layer can become very thick and may contract, squeezing the implant. When this happens, the breast tends to become hard and more round in appearance, causing discomfort or pain. If

a capsular contracture occurs, further surgery will be
required to remove the scar tissue and a new implant
may then be inserted.

Compared with implants which are placed above the chest
muscle, those placed beneath the chest muscle seldom bottom
out, and have the lowest risk of both rippling and capsular contracture.

Overall, the sub-muscular option gives the best result, but it is
the most difficult to perform and, therefore, not all surgeons are
able to offer it; it also involves the most post-op discomfort and
longest recovery time.[68]

There has recently been concern raised about the possibility of breast implants increasing the risk of breast cancer, but
there is good evidence that there is no such increased risk.[69]
However, there is some anecdotal evidence to suggest that
breast implants may be linked to a rare tumour of the immune
system called 'anaplastic large cell lymphoma' (ALCL)
which has been found, rarely, in the breast tissue around the
implants. In 2021, the European Commission and its Scientific
Committee on Health, Environmental and Emerging Risks
(SCHEER) reported that the incidence of BIA-ALCL is considered low, varies by implant type and is mainly associated with
macro-textured implants.[70]

Tissue-flap reconstruction

A tissue-flap reconstruction uses tissue from another part of the
body to reconstruct the breasts. The surgeon takes skin, fat and
sometimes muscle (a flap), typically from the abdomen or back,
and makes it into a breast shape. The surgeon will determine
which method is best based on the patient's body type and their
medical and surgical history.

It is possible to have a flap reconstruction at the same time
as the mastectomy or as a delayed reconstruction. Tissue flap

reconstruction may suit women who wish to avoid implants and who want a softer and more realistic result than a silicone implant would give.

There are various techniques that can be used during this type of reconstruction, but the most common include:

- using a muscle from the back (a latissimus dorsi flap);
- using a muscle from the abdomen (a TRAM flap);
- taking just skin and fat from the abdomen (a DIEP flap).

Each of these techniques is well described in relation to breast cancer in general on websites and in hospital leaflets so will not be covered here in detail.

Women who have had their nipple and areola complex removed during mastectomy, such as in simple mastectomy or skin-sparing mastectomy, may choose to have tattoos added to simulate breast areolae or have the skin reshaped to form a nipple. These are highly effective and often look very close to the real thing. Some women are highly creative in their choice of tattoos and may have flowers tattooed across their chests instead of nipples.

Risks associated with mastectomy and/or reconstruction

The most common complications associated with a risk-reducing mastectomy are reduced rotational movement of the shoulder, numbness of the breast and pain. Less common complications may include infection, bleeding and skin-flap necrosis (tissue death) which may require further surgery to resolve, postural changes, psychological implications and chronic pain.

16.
Survival impact – efficacy of risk-reducing surgery and breast screening on reducing cancer mortality

A study published in 2010 compared the theoretical efficacy of risk-reducing surgery with breast screening on reducing cancer mortality in 1,000,000 (one million) female BRCA1 and BRCA2 mutation carriers.[71] Researchers analysed the efficacy of no intervention, annual mammograms plus MRI from ages 25 to 69 years, risk-reducing mastectomy at various ages, and/or risk-reducing salpingo-oophorectomy at the ages of 40 or 50 years. Please note that this study was based on computer prediction models and not actual measured outcomes.

For those women who chose no intervention, researchers found that the likelihood of a 25-year-old woman surviving to the age of 70 without screening or medical interventions to prevent cancer was 53% for BRCA1 and 71% for BRCA2 mutation carriers, compared with a typical woman who has an 84% chance of surviving to the age of 70, as shown in Table 5.

Table 5: Percentage survival in women undergoing no screening or medical intervention

Group	Percentage surviving to age 70
BRCA1 mutation	53%
BRCA2 mutation	71%
Typical woman	84%

In other words, almost one in two BRCA1 mutation carriers might not live to the age of 70. The chances of surviving to the age of 70 for BRCA2 mutation carriers was higher than for BRCA1; however, it was still 13 percentage points lower than normal. Clearly, these data indicate the need for BRCA mutation carriers to have some form of screening or intervention to prevent cancer, and to improve survival.

Efficacy of breast screening on reducing cancer mortality

As previously mentioned, a 25-year-old woman with no mutation in her BRCA genes has an 84% probability of surviving to the age of 70. Of those not surviving to that age, 11% are likely to die from either breast or ovarian cancer, and 89% from other causes.

In comparison, a woman with a BRCA1 mutation who has had breast screening, but no risk-reducing medical or surgical intervention, would have only a 59% chance of reaching the age of 70 (see Table 6). This is six percentage points higher than a BRCA1 carrier with no screening, but still 25 percentage points lower than normal. Of those women not surviving, 26% would die of breast cancer, 46% of ovarian cancer and 28% of other causes.

Table 6: Percentage survival in women undergoing breast screening

Group	Percentage surviving to age 70 with breast screening alone
BRCA1 mutation	59%
BRCA2 mutation	75%
Typical woman	84%

Women with BRCA2 mutations, who undergo screening but no risk-reducing medical or surgical intervention, would have only a 75% chance of reaching the age of 70, four percentage points higher than a BRCA2 carrier with no screening, but still nine percentage points lower than normal. Of those not surviving, 21% would die of breast cancer, 25% of ovarian cancer and 54% of other causes.

These data suggest that screening alone appears to improve the likelihood of survival to the age of 70, but the likelihood of surviving to at least that age can be further improved by further medical interventions, such as risk-reducing mastectomy and salpingo-oophorectomy.

Efficacy of risk-reducing surgery on reducing cancer mortality

The most effective single intervention for BRCA1 mutation carriers is risk-reducing bilateral salpingo-oophorectomy (BSO – the removal of both ovaries and fallopian tubes) at the age of 40, yielding a 15% absolute survival gain (68% versus 53%).

For BRCA2 mutation carriers, the most effective single intervention is risk-reducing mastectomy at the age of 25, yielding an 8% survival gain (79% versus 71%); postponing risk-reducing mastectomy to the age of 40 reduces the gain by 1%. Furthermore, researchers found that the combination of risk-reducing mastectomy and risk-reducing BSO at the age of 40 improved survival more than any single intervention, yielding 24% survival gain for BRCA1 and 11% for BRCA2 mutation carriers, as shown in Table 7.

Table 7: Percentage survival in BRCA mutation carrying women undergoing risk-reducing mastectomy and BSO at age 40 compared with typical women

Group	Percentage surviving to age 70
BRCA1 mutation	77%
BRCA2 mutation	82%
Typical woman	84%

For both BRCA1 and BRCA2 mutation carriers, combining risk-reducing BSO at the age of 40 with risk-reducing mastectomy at the age of 25 offers survival approaching that of women without mutations, as shown in Table 8.

Table 8: Percentage survival in BRCA mutation carrying women undergoing risk-reducing mastectomy at age 25 and BSO at age 40

Group	Percentage surviving to age 70
BRCA1 mutation	79%
BRCA2 mutation	83%
Typical woman	84%

However, postponing risk-reducing mastectomy until the age of 40, when it may prove more acceptable than at age 25, reduces survival gain by only 1-2%. Most notably, researchers found that replacing risk-reducing mastectomy with breast screening combined with risk-reducing salpingo-oophorectomy at age 40 yields only a 3-5% decrease in survival. From these findings, researchers concluded that, although risk-reducing mastectomy at the age of 25 plus risk-reducing oophorectomy at the age of 40 years maximises survival probability, substituting breast screening for risk-reducing mastectomy seems to offer comparable survival. These results may guide women with BRCA1/2 mutations in their choices between risk-reducing surgery and breast screening. However, as previously mentioned, please bear in mind that this study was based on computer prediction models and not actual measured outcomes.

17.

The importance of a healthy diet and lifestyle in cancer prevention

Healthy lifestyle choices are important to help maintain good health and wellbeing. Adopting a healthy lifestyle may help lower the risk of developing cancer and other health conditions, such as heart disease and diabetes.

Generally speaking, everyone should:

- aim to eat at least five portions of fruit and/or vegetables a day (about 2-3 cups a day);
- limit intake of red meat and processed meat (choose chicken, fish or beans more often);
- get regular exercise (at least two to three times a week);
- achieve and maintain a healthy weight;
- choose 100% wholegrain foods (whole grain breads, cereals and brown rice);
- limit 'bad' fats (saturated and trans fats which are found in red meat, cakes/biscuits, full-fat dairy products and fried foods);
- eat 'good' fats (polyunsaturated and mono-unsaturated fats which are found in olive oil, avocado, nuts and oily fish);
- limit alcohol consumption (to fewer than one drink a day for women, and two drinks a day for men);
- not smoke.

In addition to the above, avoid processed foods, wherever possible, as they tend to contain little, if any, nutrition and are high in salt and/or sugar which, if eaten in excess, are linked to poor long-term health.

Being physically active, achieving and maintaining a healthy weight and limiting alcohol may help lower the risk of breast cancer, and cancer in general. In addition, eating a healthy diet which is rich in fruit and vegetables (at least five portions per day) has been shown to provide protection against cancer in the general population.[72] However, among BRCA mutation carriers, evidence of the role of lifestyle modification in reducing breast cancer risk is limited.[73, 74] Studies have shown that regular exercise (30 minutes, three times per week), avoidance of postmenopausal obesity, reduced alcohol intake (less than one serving per day) and avoidance of long-term hormone therapy can lead to decreased breast cancer in high-risk women.[74]

Currently, in the UK, BRCA mutation carriers are advised to eat a healthy diet which is high in fibre, low in saturated fats, which includes plenty of fruit and vegetables, to limit their alcohol intake and to participate in regular exercise. However, given the very high risk of cancer in BRCA mutation carriers, the opinion held by many is that no lifestyle or dietary factors seem to provide sufficient protection.

Although there has been a lot of research looking into the effect of dietary factors on ovarian cancer risk, so far most of the findings have been inconclusive. Some studies suggest that a diet high in animal fats may increase the risk of ovarian cancer. Furthermore, vegetables such as broccoli, cabbage and onions may decrease ovarian cancer risk but the evidence is uncertain.[75]

Since not all BRCA mutation carriers develop cancer, other factors must be involved, but further research is required to clarify this. There is a major study ongoing in the UK, known as the Epidemiological Study of Familial Breast Cancer (EMBRACE) study, which is trying to determine which lifestyle factors may modify cancer risk. Hopefully, the findings of this study will improve our understanding as to what lifestyle changes could be adopted to help prevent cancer.

Exercise

Women who engage in regular exercise have been shown to have a reduced risk of breast cancer. The question on many people's minds is just how much exercise is needed to lower the risk? In a study published in 2003, women who engaged in the equivalent of 1.25 to 2.5 hours per week of brisk walking had an 18% decreased risk of breast cancer compared with inactive women. Brisk walking for 10 hours or more per week reduced the risk a little more.[76]

Research suggests that women who are overweight or obese after menopause have an increased risk of breast cancer.[77] Before menopause, a woman's ovaries make most of her oestrogen, and fat tissue makes only a small amount. However, after menopause most of a woman's oestrogen comes from fat tissue as the ovaries no longer produce this hormone. This increased risk of breast cancer may be due in part to the higher levels of oestrogens produced by excess fat tissue after menopause.

Among women generally, exercise and healthy weight in early life are protective against breast cancer after menopause.[78] Similarly, among women with a BRCA mutation, being physically active and having had a healthy body weight as an adolescent together reduces the risk for breast cancer. A study published in 2003 showed that physical activity and a lack of obesity as an adolescent delayed the onset of breast cancer in BRCA mutation carriers.[74, 79]

A study published in 2015 calculated how much weekly exercise could reduce fat levels enough to lower the chances of developing postmenopausal breast cancer. Researchers examined the effects of the commonly recommended 150 minutes of moderate to vigorous exercise a week on body fat measures; they then compared these effects to a doubling of that amount of activity, to 300 minutes a week, to see if more exercise had a greater effect in lowering body fat. They found that those who exercised for 300 minutes a week lost more body fat, and specifically more abdominal fat than those who were active for 150 minutes each week. While the women who exercised more saw the biggest drops in their body fat measures, those who followed the recommended amount of activity – 150 minutes each week – also reduced some of their fat. But the finding suggests that more is better and, for preventing cancer, it may take more than the recommended amount of exercise to produce a benefit. 'The exercise guidelines were developed with [heart disease] outcomes in mind,' say the study's authors, Friedenreich et al. 'So at that level, they can have an effect on blood pressure, cholesterol levels and waist circumference. But for cancer prevention, we may need to exercise at higher volumes. So, yes, doing 150 minutes of activity a week is good but, if you can do more, then, from a cancer prevention perspective, 300 minutes is better.'[80, 80a]

The American Cancer Society recommends that everyone should stay at a healthy weight throughout their life by balancing food intake with physical activity and avoiding excessive weight gain. To reduce the risk of breast cancer, the American Cancer Society recommends that adults get at least 150 minutes of moderate intensity, or 75 minutes of vigorous intensity, activity each week (or a combination of these), preferably spread throughout the week.[81]

Alcohol consumption

Drinking alcohol can increase the probability of developing cancer. While there may be a perception that the health risks of alcohol only apply to heavy drinkers, research is revealing that it's not just drinking large amounts of alcohol that increases the chance of developing cancer – drinking small amounts can be harmful too.

According to Cancer Research UK, alcohol increases the risk of several cancers, including mouth, pharynx (throat), larynx (voice box), oesophagus, bowel, liver and breast cancers. There's also some evidence of an association with pancreatic cancer.[82] Generally speaking, the more alcohol you drink, the higher the likelihood of developing cancer.

Alcohol has the potential to cause cancer because it damages our DNA. A study published in 2011 found that alcohol is responsible for around 4% of UK cancers – that is, about 12,800 cases per year.[83] The proportion of cases attributable to alcohol consumption was highest for mouth and throat cancers (a little over 30%), but bowel and breast cancers accounted for the greatest overall number of cases linked to alcohol – together they accounted for about 7700 cases in 2010 (or 62% of all alcohol-related cancers). How and why alcohol increases the risk of breast cancer isn't fully understood, but one theory is that drinking alcohol affects women's hormone levels, increasing the amount of oestrogen in the body, which may fuel the growth of breast cancer.[84]

Given that alcohol increases a woman's chance of developing breast cancer in the general population, researchers have attempted to evaluate whether a similar association exists among high-risk women. With at least one exception,[85] which concluded that women with BRCA2 mutations may be at greater risk of alcohol-induced breast cancer, evidence suggests that higher risk women are not at increased risk from moderate alcohol consumption.[86, 87, 88, 89, 90]

Currently in the UK, given that alcohol is known to increase the risk of developing cancer in the general population, women with a family history of breast cancer are informed that alcohol may increase their risk slightly and they are, therefore, recommended to drink in moderation. However, given that the incidence of heart disease is higher than breast cancer and modest alcohol consumption is associated with reduced risk of heart disease, this should, according to the NICE guideline on familial breast cancer, be considered in conjunction with any potential benefit it may provide.[91]

Smoking

Cigarette smoking exposes smokers to thousands of chemicals, many of which are carcinogenic – that is, they have the potential to cause cancer. According to Cancer Research UK, smoking increases the risk of at least 14 cancers including lung cancer, cancers of the larynx (voice box), oesophagus (food pipe), mouth and pharynx (throat), bladder, pancreas, kidney, liver, stomach, bowel, cervix, ovary, nose, sinuses and some types of leukaemia, and smoking accounts for more than one in four UK cancer deaths, and nearly a fifth of all UK cancer cases.[92]

The chemicals in cigarette smoke can damage our DNA, including the DNA of genes which protect us against cancer. It is the accumulation of damage in the same cell over a period of time that can lead to cancer. Given that the repair of damage may be impaired in people with mutations in the BRCA1 or BRCA2 gene, carriers are advised not to smoke.[91]

There is also some evidence that smoking could increase the risk of breast cancer. Generally speaking, smoking is linked to a higher risk of breast cancer in younger, premenopausal women and research has also shown that there may be a link between very heavy second-hand smoke exposure and breast cancer risk in postmenopausal women.[93] In addition to the increased cancer risk, smoking can also increase complications from breast cancer treatment, including damage to the lungs from radiation therapy, difficulty healing after surgery and a higher risk of blood clots when taking hormonal replacement therapy.

Research into the effect of cigarette smoking on breast cancer risk in BRCA mutation carriers is inconsistent. Some evidence suggests that smoking does not appear to be a risk factor for breast cancer among individuals with a BRCA mutation.[94, 95] However, a later update to one of these studies found a significant positive association for BRCA1 carriers who had at least six pack-years of smoking, but who no longer smoked. ('Pack years' are the number of packets of cigarettes smoked per day multiplied by the number of years of smoking – for example, six pack-years could be one pack a day for six years or even six packs a day for one year.)[96] And, a study published in 2008 suggested that smoking is associated with increased risk of breast cancer before the age of 50 years in BRCA1 and BRCA2 mutation carriers and estimated that the risk of breast cancer increases for each pack-year.[97]

If indeed smoking is a risk factor for breast cancer for BRCA mutation carriers, then choosing not to smoke could be one of the practical ways for carriers to reduce their risks. Furthermore, a large study published in 2016, of more than 20,600 women with breast cancer, found that those who quit smoking after their diagnosis had a 33% lower risk for dying of breast cancer than those who continued to smoke.[98]

With regard to ovarian cancer, evidence suggests that there is no association between smoking and the risk of serous ovarian cancer, the type of ovarian cancer typically seen in BRCA mutation carriers. However, evidence does suggest that smoking increases the risk for the non-serous subtypes of ovarian cancer, not associated with BRCA gene mutations.[99]

In addition, a study published in 2014 confirms a vulnerability to lung cancer, a malignancy with an anticipated very poor outcome, can be inherited and implicates the BRCA2 gene as harbouring one of the involved genetic mutations.[100] The genomes of more than 11,000 individuals of European descent were scanned to look for common mutations associated with non-small cell carcinoma, a common form of lung cancer. The analysis showed that mutations in the BRCA2 and CHEK2 genes can significantly increase an individual's risk for lung cancer. The BRCA2 mutation c.9976A>T represents by far the strongest genetic association in lung cancer reported so far, as well as an increased risk for breast cancer.[100, 101] For a smoker carrying this mutation, the risk of developing lung cancer is approximately doubled. Further research is needed to see if other mutations in BRCA2 increase the risk of developing lung cancer. If it is so, then anyone known to have a mutation in this gene that is also a smoker should stop smoking based on a high risk for the development of lung cancer.

18.
Other useful information

Can children have a BRCA gene test?

Children under the age of 18 cannot usually be tested for a BRCA gene mutation. The reason for this is that they need to be old enough to decide for themselves whether or not they want to be tested. They also need to be able to understand fully all of the different implications that having the test might have for them and their family members. Furthermore, even if they were tested and were found to carry a harmful mutation, there would be no medical interventions available to them at this stage in their lives.

The major decision to be made at the age of 18 is whether or not they would wish to be aware that they carry a BRCA gene mutation at such a young age. Whilst a negative result would be very reassuring, a positive result would likely be difficult, not only because of the stress and anxiety that being aware of carrying a mutation would cause, but also because no screening would be offered until they were significantly older.

Insurance and genetic tests

Currently, there is an agreement in place between the Association of British Insurers (ABI) and the Government, known as the Concordat and Moratorium on Genetics and Insurance, which guarantees that anyone who has had a predictive genetic test (such as for breast and ovarian cancer) can take out life and critical illness insurance cover without disclosing the results.[102]

According to this agreement, people are not required to disclose the results of predictive genetic tests for policies up to £500,000 of life insurance, or £300,000 for critical illness insurance, or paying annual benefits of £30,000 for income protection insurance (the 'financial limits'). Likewise, if you already have an insurance policy in place and undergo genetic testing after your policy has started, you do not have to disclose the results for as long as the policy is in force. Furthermore, you will not be required to disclose predictive test results of family members. However, insurance companies can still ask about family history and may charge more for families with a strong family history of cancer.

According to the ABI, people who are seeking insurance will not be asked, or put under any pressure, to take a genetic test when applying for insurance. However, if you take a genetic test and you are found not to carry a mutation, you may want to tell an insurance company about these results. Many insurance companies will take this result into account, and it could counteract the effect of an unfavourable family medical history on your premium.

For further information, please see www.abi.org.uk, or your own country's Association of Insurers, or equivalent, if you do not reside in the UK.

Organ donation

BRCA mutation carriers may question if they are eligible to be an organ donor, given their BRCA status and/or personal history of cancer. However, according to the NHS Organ Donation site, there are only two conditions where organ donation is ruled out completely. A person cannot become an organ or tissue donor if they have been diagnosed with HIV (unless it is to a recipient who has HIV) or if they have, or are suspected of having, CJD (Creutzfeldt-Jakob disease), a rare, degenerative and invariably fatal brain disorder.[103]

Even though cancer may be passed from donor to recipient, in some cases organs from deceased donors with some present and past cancers may be safely used, with surgeons balancing the risk of using an organ against the risk of a patient dying waiting for a transplant. At the time that organ/tissue donation is being considered, the family would be asked about any history of cancer, the medical records would be reviewed and the family doctor would compile a report, although this is not always available pre-transplantation.

If the potential donor was confirmed as having a genetic predisposition to cancer, such as a BRCA mutation, this would be reported as part of the assessment process pre-donation and would be included as part of the information provided to the transplant surgeon. A decision would then be made by a healthcare professional, at the time of death, about whether or not the organs can be used. For further information, or if you reside in the UK and would like to become an organ donor, please visit www.organdonation.nhs.uk.

The future

Gene therapy

A powerful tool, known as 'CRISPR-Cas9' or 'CRISPR' for short, has the potential to eliminate genetic disease by making changes to our DNA which can then be passed down to future generations.

CRISPR can be thought of as a pair of molecular scissors guided by a 'molecular sat-nav' which can cut out a precise point in the DNA so that a healthy gene can then be inserted in its place. It might one day be possible to use this technique to correct a harmful mutation in the BRCA genes and to stop someone from inheriting that predisposition to breast, ovarian and prostate cancer.[104]

However, germ-line genome editing is highly controversial, even for medical purposes, with the worries it raises about 'playing God' and 'designer babies'. Currently, such modification is banned in the UK and US, but one day that may change. Many scientists believe that genetically modifying human embryos crosses an ethical line and that it should remain taboo. And, while tools such as CRISPR are incredibly powerful and simple to use, how safe it is, and how it should be used, are not yet clear.[105]

CRISPR co-developer, Professor Jennifer Doudna, and her team from the University of California, 'strongly discourage' any attempts at germ-line modification therapy that would produce genome-edited humans while the social and ethical implications are considered. They are calling for an international meeting to consider the appropriate way forward for use.[104] The other CRISPR co-developer, Professor Emmanuelle Charpentier, has also expressed her concerns to BBC News about the use of the technology to edit embryos that would then be allowed to develop into babies, and so have a permanently altered genome.[106]

Section V

My personal journey

The following chapters detail my personal journey from referral to a genetic counsellor through to my undergoing a risk-reducing bilateral salpingo-oophorectomy (BSO) and a bilateral nipple-sparing mastectomy to reduce my lifetime risk of developing breast and ovarian cancer.

I describe, openly and honestly, how I felt during these times, both physically and emotionally, as well as the effects, if any, that these operations have had on my body image, identity and sexual functioning. What follows is my own experience which may, or may not be, the experience of other women.

19.
Diagnosis and decision making

My referral for genetic counselling

After learning that my sister carried a BRCA2 gene mutation, I visited my family doctor to discuss the possibility of undergoing genetic testing myself. She explained that, in the light of this new information, I now met the 'NICE' (the UK's National Institute for Clinical Excellence) guidelines and qualified for referral for BRCA gene testing. She wrote a referral to the Genetics Department of North West Thames Regional Genetics Service in Harrow, Middlesex, England and, within a couple of weeks, I received a letter enclosing a family medical history questionnaire for my completion. I completed and returned it immediately, in the hope that I would receive an appointment to discuss testing as quickly as possible.

Within only a couple of weeks I received a 'phone call asking if I could attend at very short notice for an appointment on 5 February 2013. This was my birthday and, on this day of all days, I felt reluctant to have to face this. But, at the same time, I wanted to go through the process as quickly as possible to avoid prolonging my worry. I accepted the appointment and 'phoned my husband to inform him so that he could arrange time off work. From the very start of my journey, my husband said that he wanted to attend every appointment with me so that, no matter what was to come, we would get through it together.

The initial consultation

After arriving for my appointment, we were introduced to one of the genetic counsellors within the department and she explained that a genetic family tree had been drawn up describing how my family members were related to each other, along with any medical conditions they had from the information I had provided on my family questionnaire. She went through my family history in detail and was particularly interested in hearing my reasons for wanting to have BRCA gene testing to determine if I fully understood the implications of a positive test result.

I explained that while my mum had never been tested for a BRCA gene mutation, in all likelihood she must have been a carrier, given her diagnosis of ovarian cancer and the presence of a mutation in my sister. If my mum had indeed carried this mutation then this meant that I also had a 50:50 chance of being a carrier. I explained that this knowledge wasn't something that I could simply put to the back of my mind and do nothing about. I needed to determine if I was a carrier and, if so, I would then have the option of taking control over my future health. I mentioned that I also needed to know whether my children were at any risk; if I were found to be free of the mutation then so would my children be but, if I was a carrier, then they too would have a 50:50 chance of being carriers.

I spoke about my mum's battle with ovarian cancer and how hard it had been to see her living through this. I explained that I did not ever want to be diagnosed with ovarian cancer in my lifetime, or to die in the same way as my mum. I wanted to be there for my children, to see them grow up, graduate from university, get married and to one day have families of their own. Above all, I explained, I didn't ever want my children to have to live through their mother having cancer.

The genetic counsellor went through the pros and cons of having a genetic test, including the emotional and psychological impact that a positive genetic test result might have on me, and the implications of the result for my children. I reassured her that I was strong enough to cope with whatever the results revealed and that, if I were found to be a carrier, I would feel incredibly lucky to know about it and to then be empowered to alter the course of my destiny. After talking at considerable length the genetic counsellor agreed to my being tested and asked if I would like the blood test to be carried out at the end of the appointment. I was surprised to be offered it so soon, but I was happy to go ahead. I had wondered for many years whether I carried a BRCA gene mutation and here was my opportunity to find out, one way or another. I was ready for this.

She explained that the results would most likely be available within a few weeks, hopefully in time for her next clinic. I was sent in the direction of the phlebotomy department for the blood test. I started to feel nervous and part of me questioned if things were moving faster than I was comfortable with but, at the same time, I knew it was the right decision. If I carried this mutation, I wanted to know about it as quickly as possible and to be able to do something about it.

Waiting for my results over the next few weeks was tough – the waiting in limbo, wondering what the test would reveal and wondering what choices I would make if I were found to be a carrier. However, with being so busy raising a young family, I had very little time to spend worrying. What will be, will be, I thought.

Results day

Exactly a month after my initial appointment, the day arrived for me to collect my results. I felt a strong sense of dread and heavy-heartedness that took me back to how I had felt during my mum's illness. I wondered whether I would hear good or bad news but, whatever the case, I just wanted to know now one way or the other.

Arriving at the hospital, I said to my husband, 'Either way, this is a huge day that we will never forget.' He nodded, held my hand and smiled to reassure me. Whatever the results revealed, I knew that something positive would come – if I tested negative I would no longer need to worry, and if I tested positive I could begin the process of protecting my future health.

Whilst in the waiting room I spotted the genetic counsellor at the reception desk. I could see a concern on her face as she was looking over at me – I knew then that it wouldn't be good news. She called my name and I nervously followed her into the consulting room. Sitting in the chair, I heard the words, 'I'm so sorry you have been found to carry the same mutation as your sister.' I nodded, confirming that I had expected the result to be positive. I lowered my head, deep in thought, trying to process the words that I had just heard. Time seemed to slow down and I was in shock. I felt winded by the gravity of my results but, perhaps surprisingly, I didn't cry.

I immediately feared that I would die in the same way as my mum. I found myself imagining being in my 40s with cancer, dying in a hospice with my children next to my bedside, like her. At the same time, I feared for the future health of my two children and imagined them developing cancer and dying. My eyes began to water; this was all too much to bear. I took a deep breath, trying to hold back my tears. I looked over to my husband, almost for reassurance, but he too was clearly stunned.

Seeing that I was lost for words, my husband took the lead and asked the genetic counsellor if the best way forward was to undergo the risk-reducing surgeries. She confirmed that this is one possible option and that, if this was my decision, then the recommendation would be for them to be completed by the age of 40, as it is at that age that the incidence of BRCA-associated cancers rises sharply. She went on to explain that, in her experience, those women who have a high incidence of breast cancer within their family tend to opt for risk-reducing mastectomy (often describing it as a 'no-brainer' and that they will 'do anything to avoid chemotherapy'), whereas women with a low family history of breast cancer tend to opt for breast screening. However, in her experience, most women started with screening and some of them might at a later date opt for risk-reducing mastectomy as they could not cope emotionally with the possibility of cancer arising between screening periods. With regard to ovarian cancer, she explained, because there was no effective screening that would detect early signs of ovarian cancer and because the prognosis for the disease was poor, women tended to opt for risk-reducing BSO more readily, especially older women and those who had completed their families.

I wondered how I would ever get through it all, especially having young children and no family to support us. But, I told myself to take one step at a time, one day at a time and to try my best to remain strong throughout. I reflected on the past and how I had come through other very difficult times in my life, shaping me into the person that I was today. Somehow, I reassured myself, I would get through this too. And, even amongst all of these difficult emotions, I was intrigued to see how this particular journey would change me as a person.

The genetic counsellor handed me the results and I read for myself that I carried the BRCA2 gene mutation c.5130_5133delTGTA, referred to in the literature as '5358del4'. She confirmed that statistics suggested I had approximately a 45-85% lifetime risk of breast cancer and a 10-30% lifetime risk of ovarian cancer, along with a very slightly increased risk of pancreatic cancer and melanoma (cancer of the skin).

The genetic counsellor explained that she would notify my family doctor of the results and arrange for me to have a breast MRI to check the current health of my breasts. At the same time she would refer me to a breast surgeon and a gynaecologist to discuss my options. She explained that there would be a follow-up meeting with her for further discussion of the options

available to me, and mentioned that there was a specialist counsellor available if ever I felt the need to talk to someone.

Processing my emotions

The first few weeks after finding out I carried a BRCA2 gene mutation were one of the hardest periods of time during my journey; I was in shock and terrified about the future that lay ahead.

Having to face my own mortality for the first time wasn't easy,
but it made me think through my affairs and whether everything
was in place if anything were to happen to me. My husband and
I had taken out life insurance policies after the birth of our first
child and I felt relief that these were in place. For a brief period
of time, I considered putting a funeral plan in place, to spare my
husband and children the stress of this if I were to die, but in
the end, I decided against as it felt like a step too far. I had more
immediate decisions to make and, hopefully, this way I would
be able to avoid my own funeral for as long as possible! I did,
however, feel a strong need to talk to my husband, to make sure
that he knew my wishes if anything were to happen to me. It was
painful for both of us and so much so that I almost couldn't go
through with it. But, I needed the peace of mind that he knew my
wishes. For me, going through this process and organising my
affairs played a key part in the emotional preparation needed for
the difficult journey that lay ahead.

I felt a huge weight on my shoulders and I knew that I had
a very tough road in front of me. I was frightened and overwhelmed by the decisions that, one way or the other, I needed
to make. If risk-reducing surgery was to be the right decision
for me, I wondered how I would manage to cope with all that
these surgeries would entail, whilst also raising a young family.
My children, who were only aged 6 and 3 at this time, were too
young to be able to understand what I was going through and
were still of an age where I would have to see to their every need.

However, because I wanted to protect my children as much as possible, I put on a brave face and carried on with my daily routine. To the outside world, nobody would have known what I was dealing with internally and life would have appeared as normal.

For a brief period of time, I felt frightened of this 'thing', this mutation inside my body. This emotion took me by surprise; I hadn't expected to feel this way. However, I reasoned that the mutation had been with me since the second I was conceived, it had always been a part of me and always would be.

Perhaps surprisingly, I didn't feel anger or question, 'Why me?!' I still did not feel that anyone or anything is to blame – it is simply down to our biology and the genes that we carry. The reality is that each and every one of us carries predisposition to disease, but the only difference in people with known BRCA gene mutations is that we are aware of it and with this awareness come the many challenges of how to manage it. I accepted my mutation and instead focused my energy towards learning as much as possible about BRCA to help me to make the best, and most informed, decision to reduce my risk of developing cancer.

I felt, and always will feel, incredibly lucky to know that I carried a harmful BRCA mutation and to have become aware prior to any onset of disease. Other women aren't so fortunate. At times I felt a sense of guilt being aware of my mutation and being in the fortunate position of being able to do something about it, when for my mum, and for so many other women, this hadn't been a possibility. But, whenever this emotion arose, I reassured myself that this was what my mum would have wanted for me; it is what any parent would want for their child.

It was clear to me that on an emotional level I had two possible paths ahead of me: I could fall apart and still have to face some very difficult decisions or I could remain strong and direct my energy towards making the best decision for me. I chose the latter path, but this took a lot of strength and, at times, it wasn't always easy to remain strong. Sometimes I wanted to bury my head in the sand and not have to face any of it, but I would quickly snap out of it when I reminded myself that this was a matter of life or death – *my* life and death. To bury my head now, when I had never done so before, could have cost me my life.

While I knew that my journey with BRCA wouldn't be one of the easiest or happiest points in my life, I knew that sooner or later I would come out the other side, just as I had done with other events in the past, and that waiting ahead would be happier times for me to enjoy. I reminded myself that things could always be worse – what if one of my children had been diagnosed with cancer, or what if my husband died? That would be far worse and, although what I was facing was extremely tough, I was thankful that it wasn't as bad as what life could have thrown my way. I was also thankful to be going through this process after my own family was complete – it would undoubtedly have been a far tougher journey had I learned of my mutation prior to having children.

Approaching my journey with a positive frame of mind helped me to remain strong and to put this process into some kind of perspective. I am a firm believer in the saying that 'what doesn't kill you, makes you stronger' and I believe that every experience, good or bad, teaches and enriches us in some way. I knew that my journey with BRCA would be no exception. That said, I was still very frightened of what lay ahead.

Making a decision

I needed to make a huge decision on how I would manage my risk of developing cancer. For a brief moment, I considered the possibility of doing nothing at all – after all, I might never go on to develop breast or ovarian cancer; I might be one of the lucky ones. But, the odds were very heavily stacked against me. If you knew your flight had an 85% probability of crashing, you wouldn't get on that plane! Likewise, if you knew you had an 85% risk of breast cancer, I doubt you would choose to do nothing about it.

Personally, I did not feel comfortable with breast screening throughout the course of my life for the simple reason that my risk of developing breast cancer was exceptionally high. Even if I was lucky enough for it to be caught early, I considered the fact that there were women whose cancers had been detected at an early stage who had still succumbed to their disease. Furthermore, with this option, I would always be living in fear of developing breast cancer. If I were diagnosed with it, I might be recommended to have a mastectomy at that point, along with the removal of lymph nodes, which might result in lymphoedema, a chronic condition that causes swelling when the lymphatic system is not able to drain fluid properly. In addition to this, I might also require further treatment, including radiotherapy and chemotherapy, all of which terrified me.

Finally, with regards to ovarian screening, I was advised by my genetic counsellor that there would be no screening available to me under the NHS as it was considered to be ineffective.

As far as chemoprevention was concerned, I disliked the idea of taking medications, such as tamoxifen, to lower my risk of developing breast cancer. This was partly because the side-effects experienced by people taking this drug could be extremely difficult to tolerate, causing many to stop taking it long before the five year period is up, and also partly because of the increased risk of uterine cancer. In addition, I felt that taking a low-dose oral contraceptive, which might lower my likelihood of ovarian cancer, was not the right choice either, because of the slightly increased risk of associated breast cancer. For these reasons, chemoprevention was not an option with which I was comfortable.

This left me with the possibility of risk-reducing surgery. Whilst this was the most drastic, and in no way an appealing option, it was the one which would give me the greatest reduction in risk of developing both breast and ovarian cancer. These at-risk tissues could be removed from my body, thereby lowering my risk of ovarian cancer down to approximately 1% and my risk of breast cancer down to approximately 3-5% to age 70. Being able to reduce my risks down to as low as this was phenomenal and, for me personally, it felt like the most logical step to take.

I briefly considered removing only my ovaries and fallopian tubes given that my mum developed ovarian cancer and not breast cancer. I wondered if perhaps the same would hold true for me. Then again, perhaps my mum would have gone on to develop breast cancer had she not died from ovarian cancer. I considered how removing my ovaries would approximately halve my risk of developing breast cancer – just maybe, I wondered, would removing my ovaries be enough to prevent both cancers. But, then again, even with halving my risk of breast cancer the risk would still be too high for my liking. In addition to this, if I were to remove my ovaries, I would want to take HRT to ease the menopausal symptoms and to protect my long-term health, but taking HRT would be putting back some of the oestrogen and progesterone into my body which, in turn, might again increase my risk of developing breast cancer.

I considered also how devastated I would be if I made the decision to undergo only the removal of my ovaries and tubes, hoping that the reduction in risk of breast cancer would be sufficient, only to then be diagnosed with breast cancer. With everything considered, I was not comfortable with solely removing my ovaries as a method of managing my lifetime risk of both breast and ovarian cancer.

Personally, I wanted to lower my risk of developing breast cancer and ovarian cancer by as much as possible and, for this reason, I soon knew that undergoing both risk-reducing surgeries was the right decision for me. However, an emotion which lingered for many months was this feeling of having a choice, but not *really* having a choice. I didn't want to have to have my ovaries or my breasts removed, but I knew that doing so would give me the very best protection against cancer. Very reluctantly, I began to prepare myself, mentally and emotionally, for major and life-changing surgery.

Having seen my mum suffer ovarian cancer, the decision to remove my ovaries and fallopian tubes was certainly the easier of the two decisions to make. I would do whatever it took to avoid ovarian cancer, but what was difficult was the fear of the unknown and the fear of what it might do to my health in other ways. I was terrified by the thought of undergoing surgery, whether or not I would experience any complications and what effect removing my ovaries would have on my overall health and wellbeing. I was also terrified by the idea of going through the menopause and, particularly, a surgically induced menopause, as I was aware that this could be more severe than a natural one. Until now, the menopause was something a long way off in my future and not something I had ever really given any thought to at the relatively young age of 35.

To try to prepare myself for what the menopause might bring, I read up on the possible symptoms. I wondered what it would feel like to experience hot flushes and I was worried about the possibility of insomnia. I had had years of sleep deprivation with my two children, from waking during the night or being woken up early for years on end. The thought of losing any more sleep was not at all appealing. I was also scared of the possibility of depression and, above all, I was concerned about the effect of the menopause on my sex life. I worried about the possibility of developing vaginal dryness and whether or not I would develop a loss of sensation and pleasure that some women reportedly experience after ovary removal. And, if so, would I find it harder to achieve orgasm or would I perhaps lose the ability to experience it altogether? I feared my love life might be destroyed and questioned whether I could be happy and fulfilled living a life that didn't include making love. It didn't seem fair having to worry about all of these possibilities in my 30s. I had so far enjoyed a healthy love life with my husband and I wanted it to continue.

For the first time in my life, I also started to fear the possibility of becoming overweight. I had always enjoyed a good figure and had never had to worry about my weight, or the shape of my body, in any way. But now I feared that this may change with the removal of my ovaries.

As if all of this wasn't enough to fear, just what effect would removing my ovaries have on my long-term health? While on the one hand their removal would, of course, protect my health by reducing my risk of developing ovarian and breast cancer, on the other hand it might cause harm, in terms of increasing my risk of developing osteoporosis and heart disease. While I would be preventing cancer, I might be opening the door to a number of other diseases. At that time, I was in excellent health and removing my ovaries might have jeopardised that. Once they had been removed there would, of course, be no going back.

Coming to terms with the decision to remove my breasts was an extremely difficult and emotional process. They were a very important part of my womanhood. I had only recently finished breastfeeding my youngest, which had been one of the most beautiful experiences in my life, and now to have to face removing them felt as if I was betraying them in some way, and worse still was the fear that I would feel mutilated or even violated by these surgeries. In addition, my breasts played a very important part in my love life and I wondered what effect losing them, and the erotic sensation that I would lose along with them, would have on my overall enjoyment of making love. Trying to look at the positives, however, if there was ever a right time to have to lose them, it would be after they had fulfilled their role breastfeeding my children and prior to them becoming a threat to my life.

Only naturally, I questioned whether I would feel less of a

woman without my breasts and ovaries – after all, it was these parts of my body which made me female. Fearing this as a possibility was just awful, but while this mutation could take my ovaries and breasts, it couldn't remove my XX chromosome. I figured, I am genetically female and always will be – nothing can change that. Furthermore, my husband reassured me that, in his eyes, I would be more of a woman for finding the bravery and strength to face my fate head on and to do whatever was necessary to protect our family from the trauma of cancer.

Undergoing an MRI

Whilst I was certain of my decision to undergo risk-reducing surgery, I was still eager to have a 'magnetic resonance imaging' (MRI) scan to determine the current health of my breasts.

At the start of May 2013, I underwent my first (and what was to be the only) MRI. Sitting in the waiting room, awaiting my scan, I began to feel overwhelmed with fear; fear of having the scan and, worse still, fear that a cancer would be found. If I was this scared, when as far as I knew I was in good health and was simply undergoing screening, just how scared would I be to learn that I had cancer, only to then have to face the possibility of chemotherapy and radiotherapy? In this moment I was 100% certain that a risk-reducing mastectomy was the best way forward to avoid ever having to go through any of this trauma in the future.

Awaiting my results was stressful but, to my relief, within a few days I received a 'phone call to say that my MRI was normal. The radiologist's report, which I saw much later, read:

> 'both breasts have a moderately dense glandular pattern. No focal areas of abnormal morphology or enhancement to suggest malignant disease.'

I felt incredibly lucky and, at that moment, my heart went

out to all of those women who do not receive such good news. However, given my very high lifetime risk of breast cancer, I couldn't help but feel that it would have only been a matter of time until one day the news would not have been so good.

Breast density

I only found out that my breasts were 'moderately dense' after I had undergone both risk-reducing surgeries and had requested the findings of my MRI for the purposes of writing this book. I was shocked to learn the result as, even though evidence suggests increased mammographic breast density is not associated with higher breast cancer incidence in women with BRCA mutations, breast density is nonetheless considered a risk factor for developing breast cancer overall. For this reason, I felt that I ought to have been informed at the time of my 'normal' MRI result, as is routinely done in some countries; had I been aware of this prior to undergoing my risk-reducing mastectomy, it would have further reinforced my decision.

A couple of days after receiving the results from my MRI, I heard on the news that the actress, Angelina Jolie, had undergone a risk-reducing mastectomy because of a harmful mutation in her BRCA1 gene. I could hardly believe my ears and immediately felt a sense of closeness towards her, not only because we both carried a BRCA gene mutation, but also because we have both experienced the loss of a mother to ovarian cancer. I felt great admiration and respect for her and her brave decision to share her story with the world for the benefit of other women.

Consultation with a gynaecologist

A week after my MRI scan, I attended an initial appointment with a gynaecologist. I explained that I had come to the decision to have my ovaries and fallopian tubes removed. The doctor explained that this would be the most effective option in lessening my lifetime risk of developing ovarian cancer. She asked me if I was sure that my family was complete and I assured her that I was certain of this. She recommended having this surgery around the age of 40, or sooner, and explained that this could be done laparoscopically. I explained that given my mum's diagnosis with ovarian cancer in her early 40s, I personally felt a stronger need to remove my ovaries and tubes ahead of undergoing a mastectomy. In doing so, I would reduce my risk for ovarian cancer, whilst also lessening my risk for breast cancer at the same time.

Even though screening for ovarian cancer is not routinely offered on the NHS, I explained to the gynaecologist that I was uncomfortable with the idea of having no screening at all, especially given that ovarian cancer only tends to be symptomatic in late-stage disease, by which time a patient's prognosis is poor. I explained that if there were to be a cancerous tumour on my ovaries then just maybe these screening tests would detect it at an early enough stage to improve my chances of survival. With this, she completed the paperwork for me to have an ultrasound and a CA-125 blood test and explained that I would receive a follow-up appointment with her to ask any further questions that I might have. Thankfully, the results from these tests were normal. However, given the doubt over the effectiveness of screening for ovarian cancer, I wasn't wholly reassured and I continued to feel an urgency to have my ovaries removed as quickly as possible.

Follow-up with the genetic counsellor

A couple of months after my MRI scan and gynaecology appointment, I returned to the hospital for my follow-up appointment with the genetic counsellor.

During this meeting, I explained that I had since had a breast

MRI, a pelvic ultrasound and a CA-125 blood test and that all of these were normal. I explained that I had made a decision to have my ovaries and tubes removed and also to undergo a risk-reducing mastectomy because it was this option which would offer me the very best protection against developing breast and ovarian cancer.

I explained that, even with the support of my husband and friends, I felt very alone. Ultimately, it was me that would have to go through these surgeries, the menopause and any consequences to my overall health. The genetic counsellor reassured me that it was common for people to feel alone on this journey and, again, she offered the services of the specialist psychologist who would be there to support me through any of my emotions. I confirmed that for now I was coping well, but that if this were to change then I would certainly make use of this service in future.

Having made the decision to undergo risk-reducing surgery, it was again recommended that I do so by around 40 years of age, or sooner if I was certain that my family was complete. The genetic counsellor also explained that undergoing a salpingo-oophorectomy would result in me becoming sterile, meaning that I would be unable to produce any more children. This fact was clear to me and, being blessed with both a son and a daughter, I was not concerned by the prospect of becoming sterile. However, I imagine that this decision would be a painful one for women without children, or for women without the same certainty that their family was complete; I could only be thankful that this wasn't the case for me personally.

The genetic counsellor also recommended that I have a bone density scan before removing my ovaries so that they could monitor my bone density thereafter, as one of the problems with early menopause was osteoporosis. I was also reminded of the importance of eating a healthy diet that was rich in calcium and vitamin D, and to undertake regular exercise to help maintain my health and to prevent osteoporosis and heart disease. I reassured her that I had always eaten a very healthy diet and regularly exercised, and that I would continue to do so.

I mentioned that, ideally, I wanted to discuss my options with more than one specialist, as it was important for me to determine that the information I was being given was consistent between doctors of the same specialty. The decisions that I was facing were major and life-changing and I needed the peace of mind that these were founded on sound medical advice. I was reassured that, under the NHS, it would, indeed, be possible for me to get a second opinion.

Consultation with a breast surgeon

A couple of days after my follow-up appointment with the genetic counsellor, and nearly four months after learning of my BRCA mutation, I had my first NHS appointment with a breast surgeon.

I explained that I had decided to have a risk-reducing mastectomy, preferably with immediate reconstruction with implants, so that the mastectomy and reconstruction could be combined into one surgical procedure. He wholly supported my decision, explaining that it would be the most effective option for lessening my risk of developing breast cancer. I also explained that it was important for me to have reconstruction, preferably with implants, as I disliked the idea of alternative methods, such as the DIEP flap as it would be more invasive, leaving me with more scarring and a longer recovery time. He agreed that reconstruction with implants would be a good option for me as in his opinion I had too little body fat for a DIEP flap to be performed.

For this type of reconstruction, he recommended that an 'acellular dermal matrix' be used. This is an animal skin which provides an additional layer of tissue between the skin and the implant which helps to provide a much more natural shape to the reconstructed breast. This matrix has been processed to make it completely safe to use in humans.

I mentioned that I would prefer to have a nipple-sparing

mastectomy in order to keep my breasts looking as close in appearance to my natural breasts as possible. As far as I had been able to determine from my own reading, this was an acceptable choice for patients with BRCA mutations, with no evidence of compromise to oncological safety. However, he questioned the possibility of a theoretical risk leaving the nipple intact and his recommendation was, therefore, to remove both nipples. This was really difficult for me to hear; I felt on the verge of tears. The nipples are perhaps the most important and defining part of a woman's breast. Considering losing them felt much harder emotionally than leaving them intact. But, I thought, if this was what would be best, if this was what evidence suggested would give me the greatest reduction in risk, then I would, ultimately, have my nipples removed.

The breast surgeon went on to explain that, if I chose to proceed with a nipple-sparing mastectomy, I would need to be referred to a different surgeon as he personally was not experienced in performing this kind of procedure.

I found it particularly hard to keep my wits about me during this appointment; discussing the removal of my breasts and possibly my nipples along with them was horrendous. I battled with myself internally to stay focused and to take in what I was being told, but, emotionally, it was all too much. For this reason, I was glad to have someone attend the appointment with me, as not only was my husband a great source of support, he was also able to absorb some of the information that had washed over me.

While attending this appointment in itself was helpful, the next couple of weeks that followed were particularly difficult. The process of removing my breasts now felt all the more real and I was devastated.

A week or so later, to try to alleviate my stress levels and to avoid the NHS waiting times, I decided to book a private appointment with a further breast surgeon who had been highly recommended to me. He had many years' experience, which I felt immediately reassured by, and I was eager to gain his opinion on what I should do for the best with regard to removing my nipples. His recommendation to me was to undergo a nipple-sparing mastectomy. He explained that while there is a theoretical risk to the nipple, it was highly unlikely. In addition to this, I also felt very reassured that, in his personal experience, none of the women who had undergone a nipple-sparing mastectomy had returned with breast cancer in the years following their surgery.

He mentioned that the current recommendations are for BRCA mutation carriers to undergo risk-reducing mastectomy 10 years before the earliest diagnosed case of BRCA-associated cancer within their family (and in the case of oophorectomy, so long as their family is complete). Given that my mum's ovarian cancer was at 44 years old, and that there were no other cases, the recommendation for me personally was for surgery to be done around the age of 34. I was already aged 35 and had, therefore, just entered into this period in time.

He went on to explain that he would be happy to perform my surgery, although he was due to retire imminently. He recommended his colleague, Mr Tyler, a consultant plastic and reconstructive surgeon, at Stoke Mandeville Hospital, England, whom he described as 'the best' and explained that he would write to him after our meeting. However, while he was described to me as the best, there are, of course, many other excellent surgeons working within the NHS.

Consultation with another breast surgeon

A couple of months later, I had my first appointment with Mr Tyler. I explained that I had decided to have a mastectomy with immediate reconstruction with implants, ideally using the acellular dermal matrix that had been recently recommended to me. He asked to examine me and confirmed that I would be a very good candidate for implants for the reasons that my breasts were quite small, my nipples were well positioned on my breasts (i.e. they did not point downwards), there was a small amount of loose skin from having breastfed and I had not had any prior surgery or radiation to this area.

He explained that he would use a silicone implant, but I raised my concerns over their quality and safety. I was aware of the reported problems with PIP implants which had been fraudulently manufactured using unapproved silicone gel, making them far more prone to splitting (rupturing) than other breast implants. However, he reassured me that the PIP implants had all been withdrawn from the UK and the implants that he would use are safe and of a very good quality. This put my mind at rest, but I continued to feel uncomfortable at the idea of having implants within my body as they simply aren't natural. But, at the same time, having some form of breast reconstruction was important to me and, with the alternatives appealing even less, reconstructing with implants was, for me personally, my only option.

Touching on the topic of removing or retaining my nipples, his recommendation was to undergo a nipple-sparing mastectomy, for the reason that evidence does not suggest that retaining the nipple compromises oncological safety. I was very relieved that this was his recommendation and, from this moment onwards, my decision was to proceed in this way. I was, however, keen to determine if he had known of any patients throughout the course of his career, or any of his colleagues' careers, who had undergone a nipple-sparing mastectomy and had at a later date presented with breast cancer; I was relieved to hear that he had not.

He then explained the different types of incision that could be used to perform the mastectomy, including making an incision on the side of the breast, or through the nipple-areola complex, or through the infra-mammary fold (IMF). He felt that he would most likely go through the nipple which, he explained, would leave me with small, but visible, scarring. I found the idea of being left with visible scarring over the front of my breast difficult to come to terms with and it took many months before I felt at peace with this.

We discussed the possible complications of a mastectomy, including the risk of bleeding and infection, both of which might result in further surgery and subsequent implant loss. However, he explained that the risk of infection would be reduced with a two-week course of antibiotics starting immediately after the procedure. He mentioned that approximately 10% of patients who undergo a mastectomy develop necrosis (tissue death). He explained that when the breast tissue is removed, some of the nerves and blood vessels are also unavoidably removed and, if inadequate blood flow remains to the skin, it can lead to the tissue dying as a result of too little oxygen reaching the tissues. If this were to happen, further surgery would be necessary to resolve the issue, which might also result in loss of the implant(s). However, he reassured me that given that my breasts were quite small, that I was healthy and a non-smoker with no underlying diseases, such as diabetes (both of which might cause poor circulation and, thus, a higher risk of necrosis), he felt that the risk of this particular complication in my case would, hopefully, be low.

He explained that I would most likely lose sensitivity in my breasts, including the loss of the erotic sensation. He also wanted me to understand that I might require further surgery at some point in the future, as the implants and/or acellular dermal matrix might not last a lifetime and might, therefore, need replacing. The thought of future surgery wasn't appealing, but whatever would be, would be, I thought.

Raising my fear of how painful it would be to undergo a mastectomy, he reasoned that while it was likely to feel quite uncomfortable, any pain would hopefully be effectively managed with pain relief, both during my hospital stay and post-discharge. He explained that after waking from surgery, I would have patient-controlled anaesthesia (PCA) containing morphine which I could access for pain relief as often as required. Upon discharge, I would be sent home with more standard painkillers, such as paracetamol and ibuprofen. With this, I felt a little more reassured, but continued to fear just how painful this surgery would be.

During this period of time, I had been saddened by the thought that I would no longer be able to wear beautiful lingerie, instead resigning myself to specially designed mastectomy bras or, perhaps, t-shirt bras. I imagined that these wouldn't be as attractive or as sexy as the bras I had so far enjoyed wearing. However, thankfully, I was mistaken and he reassured me that once I had fully recovered from surgery (after around six to eight weeks), I should be able to wear any bra, including those that are under-wired. I could now look forward to the day, post-surgery, when I could treat myself to some new bras.

A further concern of mine was the mastectomy interfering with my ability to exercise. I was aware that some women reportedly develop a reduced rotational movement of the arm. However, Mr Tyler reassured me that, once fully recovered, I should be able to exercise as before and that, if necessary, I would be given some physiotherapy to resolve any such difficulties. He went on to reassure me further, explaining that there was nothing that I wouldn't be able to do once fully recovered and, to my surprise, he even mentioned that the implants are so tough that they could withstand being stood on! Given their durability, I felt confident that having implants wouldn't affect my ability to lead a normal life.

Visit to an early menopause clinic

To learn more about the symptoms of menopause, and to discuss hormone-replacement therapy (HRT), I was referred to an early menopause clinic held at Northwick Park Hospital, London, UK.

I met with one of the specialist nurses and shared with her my concern over the effect that removing my ovaries would have on my love life and, to a lesser extent, on my figure. She explained that the menopause can lead to weight gain, but reassured me that younger women who go through the menopause do not tend to experience this in the same way that older women do. The possibility of weight gain tends to be an age-related issue, she explained, which is related to lifestyle factors, such as a poor diet or a lack of exercise. If women eat healthily and exercise regularly, they will be less likely to gain weight. Furthermore, she reassured me that so long as a woman was receiving an adequate dose of HRT, removing the ovaries would not lead to a reduction in metabolism and, hence, weight gain.

I wanted to know whether my ability to have an orgasm would be affected after ovary removal. She reassured me that it is stimulation to the upper third of the vagina and the cervix which are important for orgasm, and not the ovaries. While I knew this to be true, I couldn't help but fear whether removing the ovaries might, in some way, have an impact on this. However, she explained that some women who have had their cervix/uterus removed might experience a significant loss in sexual arousal and ability to orgasm during intercourse.

I mentioned that I was struggling to decide whether or not to have my uterus removed. She explained that, in her experience, women often find this decision to be a difficult one. While she highlighted the importance of making the right decision for me personally, from her point of view in her role as a menopause nurse, it could be more challenging to manage the menopause in women who kept their uterus. The reason for this was that these women would then need to take a combined HRT, containing both oestrogen and progesterone; the progesterone, she warned, can bring on PMT-like symptoms which some women find un-pleasant and difficult to manage. However, if I were to have my uterus removed, I would be able to take oestrogen-only HRT and would be unlikely to experience these symptoms. In addition, she explained that the risk of breast cancer with oestrogen-only HRT might be more favourable than with combined HRT, making the decision especially hard for women who had not chosen risk-reducing mastectomy. However, in such cases, she explained, this would need to be offset against the potential risks of hysterectomy and, therefore, a full discussion with a gynaecologist would be essential.

I raised my concern over what effect the menopause would have on my mental, emotional and physical wellbeing. I feared that it would turn me into an irritable, anxious, moody and perhaps even a depressed person. Ultimately, I was terrified that I would have some kind of personality transplant, turning me into an entirely different person. However, she reassured me that there are women who breeze through the menopause, with little or no difficulty, and that I might be one of them. But, if not, she explained, the HRT would normally be very effective in helping manage the symptoms. It might take a few months to get me on the right dose or the right kind of HRT before the symptoms settled down but, she reassured me, eventually it would get me back to the person that I was now.

Finally, I questioned whether removing my ovaries and becoming menopausal would accelerate the ageing of my skin and hair. Here she put my mind to rest by explaining that while the menopause affects skin and hair over time, taking HRT would help to prevent these changes. Furthermore, she explained that women going through the menopause at the usual age of around 50 are the most affected as they have combined ageing effects too which are probably of equal significance. She also concluded that in all women good skin care, eating a healthy diet and leading a healthy lifestyle would all help to prevent premature ageing of the skin and hair.

This meeting was very informative and it really helped to allay many of my fears about the menopause. Perhaps the most helpful of all was taking away with me the reassurance, and the peace of mind, that whatever the menopause brings I would one day get back to my normal self.

Consultation with a gynaecological oncologist

A month after my appointment at the early-menopause clinic, and now seven months after being informed of my BRCA mutation, I continued to have questions which remained unanswered, despite further follow-up appointments with the initial gynaecologist. It became clear to me that I needed to seek the expertise of a gynaecologist with a strong knowledge of BRCA-associated ovarian cancer. To try to ease my stress as quickly as possible, and to avoid waiting a couple of months for an alternative appointment, I decided to contact a private hospital, close to where I lived. I was immediately relieved, and reassured, to hear that they had a gynaecological oncologist within the hospital who had expertise in both gynaecology and oncology. In mid-October, I attended an initial appointment with Mr Drake, at the Spire Harpenden Hospital, England.

After explaining to him that I carried a BRCA2 gene mutation and that I had decided to undergo a bilateral salpingo-oophorectomy (BSO), he confirmed that this would be his recommendation to me. He reasoned that it was the most effective strategy for lowering the risk of developing ovarian cancer, a disease which he described as having a very poor prognosis. He also mentioned that, with regard to women undergoing risk-reducing mastectomy, there was plenty of psychological research showing that women who have had this surgery were far happier knowing that their risk had been properly addressed. For me, I knew that this point would also hold true for undergoing an oophorectomy; I would not be happy until my risk of both breast and ovarian cancer had indeed been properly addressed.

With regard to my uterus, he did not hold the opinion that this was at increased risk of developing cancer as a result of my BRCA gene mutation and, therefore, he recommended proceeding only with a BSO, which he explained could be performed laparoscopically. However, he warned that leaving the uterus intact would mean that a small part of the fallopian tube would inevitably be left in the outside wall of the uterus and that this would hypothetically give me a risk of tubal or primary peritoneal cancer. But he reassured me that the risk of this was extremely low and that it was certainly not a reason to dismiss risk-reducing surgery. He reassured me that what was important to know was that bilateral salpingo-oophorectomy in BRCA mutation carriers massively reduces the risk for ovarian cancer.

I wanted to find out his opinion on the possibility of sal-pingectomy with delayed oophorectomy; that is, removing both fallopian tubes but leaving both ovaries intact, for a while at least, to avoid the negative side-effects and long-term health consequences associated with oophorectomy at a young age. However, he strongly advised against this, holding the opinion that this strategy might be ineffective in reducing a woman's risk of developing ovarian cancer because the ovaries themselves might develop malignancy.

We also discussed the possibility of removing only one fallopian tube and one ovary while leaving the other side intact, again to avoid the negative side-effects and long-term health consequences associated with oophorectomy at a young age, but Mr Drake did not endorse this option either. He explained that if we removed the right fallopian tube and ovary, but cancer developed within the left tube or ovary, our attempt to lower my risk of ovarian cancer would have been totally unsuccessful. Furthermore, given that cancer which arises as a result of genetic mutations is more likely to be a bilateral cancer (that is, cancer that occurs in both of a pair of organs, such as both ovaries), removing only one ovary and one fallopian tube might not offer any significant protection against ovarian cancer. Mr Drake's advice was simple: only by removing both ovaries and both fallopian tubes would we achieve maximum, and satisfactory, risk-reduction.

As with the other surgeons, he again explained that, for those who choose to have risk-reducing surgery, the current recommendation is to undergo risk-reducing oophorectomy five to 10 years before the earliest diagnosed case of BRCA-associated cancer within their family, so long as their family is complete. He went on to explain that we could potentially delay surgery for a couple more years until I was closer to the age of 40, but he also said, 'Why wait?' He reasoned that given my certainty that my family was complete and that my mum had been diagnosed with ovarian cancer at a very young age for a BRCA2 mutation carrier, the best course of action would be to go ahead with surgery as soon as possible. I knew that his words were wise; the thought of delaying this surgery by a couple of years and the possibility of being diagnosed with cancer during that time filled me with terror.

At the end of this appointment, I felt very happy that all of my remaining questions had been answered. I now felt very well informed and confident in my decision to undergo a BSO. Given Mr Drake's outstanding expertise in both gynaecology and oncology, I trusted that I would be in the best of hands in his care and I felt confident that he was the right surgeon for me.

He explained that he would be available to perform my surgery within the next four or so weeks. The thought of having surgery so soon was unnerving but, at the same time, given that I felt that my BRCA mutation was effectively a ticking time bomb, the sooner that I had this surgery, the better.

Decision on uterus (womb) removal

Making the decision on whether or not to remove my uterus was one of the most challenging of all; it took many months of uncertainty before I finally came to a decision.

Most experts believe the risk for uterine cancer in women with BRCA mutations is similar to that of women in the general population. For that reason, the removal of the uterus, known as a hysterectomy, at the same time as BSO, is not universally recommended for carriers of a BRCA mutation.

All of the consultants that I saw held the opinion that there was no link between uterine cancer and BRCA mutations; hence, they did not recommend a hysterectomy. I trusted their opinions and particularly that of Mr Drake – after all they were highly qualified doctors. On the other hand, a doubt remained in my mind. I wondered whether, with future research, such recommendations might change. I also considered how I no longer had a need for my uterus with my family being complete, and the possibility that I could develop a sporadic uterine cancer (that is, a cancer that arises for some other reason and not as a result of a BRCA mutation). However, even with these points in mind, the specialists continued to maintain that removing my uterus was unnecessary.

I decided to take a look at the available medical literature. Confusingly, some of this research suggests that there is no link between BRCA mutations and uterine cancer, while other studies suggest that there might be a link, albeit perhaps only for BRCA1, and not BRCA2, mutation carriers. Perhaps what is true is that some BRCA mutations confer a risk for uterine cancer, while others do not. Only with continued research will the picture become clearer.

As a result, I found it difficult to know what to believe and, therefore, what to do for the best. However, given that all of the specialists that I saw held the opinion that carrying a BRCA gene mutation did not increase my risk for uterine cancer, and given that I had not come across any studies suggesting that my specific BRCA2 gene mutation confers a risk, overall, I felt reassured that it would be acceptable to keep my uterus. I was also very reassured that after my mum's surgery, her uterus was found to be entirely healthy, with no sign of cancer.

In addition to this, a hysterectomy was described to me as a more complicated operation, with a higher risk of morbidity than a BSO alone, including an increased risk of infection, bleeding during or following surgery, and/or damage to internal organs such as the urinary tract or bowel. Because the uterus provides support for the top of the vagina, there is also the possibility of a vaginal prolapse, and specifically a vaginal vault prolapse, in which the top of the vagina falls toward, and may even protrude out of, the vaginal opening. This condition is common after a hysterectomy, with more than 10% of women developing some degree of prolapse after surgery. On top of all of this, hysterectomy alone has also been associated with sexual function problems, such as a lack of lubrication and a decrease in sexual pleasure and the ability to achieve orgasm during intercourse, among others.

Clearly, there was a lot of information to absorb and a long decision-making process to go through. However, after several months of weighing everything up in my mind, I decided to keep my uterus intact.

20.
My risk-reducing surgeries

In this chapter I share with you my own experience of under-going a bilateral salpingo-oophorectomy (BSO) and bilateral nipple-sparing mastectomy with immediate reconstruction with implants. I detail, openly and honestly, the emotions I felt dur-ing and after my surgeries, along with the physical experience of undergoing surgery and the surgically induced menopause which followed the removal of my ovaries. I also share any ef-fects these operations have had on my body image, identity and sexual functioning.

Some of the thoughts and emotions that I have experienced will be common to most women who have been found to carry a harmful BRCA gene mutation, but some may be unique to me. My aim is simply to share my own journey in the hope that it may help you with yours.

Undergoing a bilateral salpingo-oophorectomy (BSO)

A few weeks after consulting Mr Drake, the consultant gynaeco-logical oncologist, and a little over eight months after learning of my BRCA2 gene mutation, the day arrived for me to undergo surgery to remove both ovaries and tubes.

Arriving at the hospital, I was greeted by the nurse who would be looking after me. After showing me to my room, she measured me up for a pair of anti-deep vein thrombosis (DVT) stockings which would help prevent the development of clots during and after surgery. She explained that she would need to carry out a pregnancy test to confirm that I wasn't pregnant. If this was found to be positive, she explained, the surgery would need to be cancelled. However, as I knew it would, the test revealed that I wasn't pregnant and the surgery could go ahead as planned.

A short while later Mr Drake arrived and kindly asked how I was feeling. I explained that I was nervous but that, nonetheless, I continued to be certain of my decision to have my ovaries removed. I also mentioned that I was scared of the menopause, particularly a surgically induced one, given that it might be more severe than a natural one. Trying to reassure me, he explained that, in his experience, some women were absolutely fine, while others could be very symptomatic, meaning they become very emotional quickly after surgery. I felt sorry for those women and wondered if this would be my reality too.

He advised that I should avoid taking HRT after surgery, until after my mastectomy, as research in general showed that the risk of breast cancer increased even within the first year of taking HRT. I felt all the more terrified of an imminent menopause which would not be in any way alleviated by HRT. However, he reassured me that if I became particularly symptomatic with disabling menopausal symptoms, then there would be little choice but to start HRT.

Mr Drake explained that he would see me again shortly, in theatre. A couple of hours later, there was a knock at my door and in walked two men dressed in theatre gowns, explaining that they were ready for me. I saw the surprise on their face that I was young and a picture of health. They asked if I needed a wheelchair, but I explained that that wouldn't be necessary. I put on my dressing gown and slippers and followed the men along the corridor.

It felt a little bizarre walking towards theatre feeling in perfectly good health, but knowing that I would be imminently undergoing surgery. Arriving at the other end of the corridor, outside the lifts down to theatre, my husband was told that he wouldn't be able to go any further. At that moment, I felt as if I would crumble into a quivering wreck. We cuddled, both of us close to tears.

In the lift, the theatre staff engaged in polite chit-chat to try to ease my anxieties, but I felt consumed by my emotions. I felt intensely vulnerable, alone and frightened. I was guided in to the pre-op room where I would be prepared for theatre. Entering the room, I was taken aback by the warmest of greetings from all of the staff who would be looking after me and I realised that this was something they do to try to ease a patient's anxieties. It worked, for a moment at least.

I was asked to remove my dressing gown and to lie down on the bed but I hesitated, fearing how I would feel when I awoke on the other side. Reluctantly, I climbed on to the bed and lay down. The theatre staff started to prepare me for surgery, while my consultant checked my name, date of birth and confirmed the surgery that I was due to undergo. I looked over at the anaesthetist and could see she was preparing the anaesthetic. Despite how warm the room felt, I started to feel very cold which I realised was due to my nerves. This quickly worsened into a trembling, which I couldn't control. My arms and upper body were shaking, more than I had ever experienced in my life before. One of the lovely theatre staff grabbed my hand to try to reassure me, while sharing with me how nervous he had been a few months previously having only his tonsils removed.

The anaesthetist explained that she would give me the pre-op medication for pain relief. I felt a little woozy, but it was a nice feeling and I felt very relaxed. Moments later, I watched the anaesthetic being administered into my cannula, despite their best efforts to keep this away from sight. I decided to close my eyes and my final thought before falling asleep was feeling pleased with myself for having come this far.

When I awoke from surgery, I was immediately aware of some discomfort from the incisions on either side of my pelvis and, particularly so on the right-hand side. (My surgeon later told me that the right side is often the sorest because it is through this incision that both ovaries are removed.) However, I was surprised that there was no discomfort in my navel where a smaller, third incision would have been made. The nurse gave me some morphine and within a couple of minutes I felt more comfortable. Otherwise, and to my complete amazement, I felt perfectly well; I could hardly believe that my body had just gone through surgery. I lay there, enjoying the sense of relief that the operation was over and, above all, the incredible feeling of being free of the worry of one day being diagnosed with ovarian cancer.

Within half an hour or so, I was wheeled back to my room on the surgical ward. I could see my husband waiting nervously. I smiled to reassure him that I was okay and I could see his worries fade away before my eyes. He too was surprised to see me looking and feeling so well. While I felt relief that the surgery was over, the fear of experiencing the menopause and what effect removing my ovaries would have on my health now felt all the more real and, perhaps only naturally, I feared that I had not done the right thing.

Within a few minutes, Mr Drake arrived, seemingly eager to reassure me that the operation had gone smoothly and that everything appeared to be normal and healthy, although he of course explained that we could only be sure of this once we had the findings of the pathology report. I understood that but, for now at least, I was very relieved.

Now that I had had the surgery, my fear of the menopause and what I might have done to my overall health was greater than ever. Mr Drake reassured me that I had made the right choice and reiterated that removing my ovaries had given me the greatest reduction in risk of developing ovarian cancer. I felt reassured, but I remained fearful of the menopause and what it had in store for me. I couldn't escape the feeling that it would be me and me alone who would ultimately have to go through it. I felt intensely alone, even with my husband at my side.

Throughout the day, I continued to be aware of the discomfort from the incisions, especially if I tried to move. My abdomen had been distended with air which was also uncomfortable. Nevertheless, I enjoyed the rare opportunity of lying down in the middle of the day – what a luxury that was!

I didn't have much of an appetite, but I had an insatiable thirst, most likely caused by the morphine. I enjoyed drinking glass after glass of water but when I asked for yet another jug of water, the nurse advised me to slow down and to only take small sips, every now and then, so as to not worsen the discomfort from my distended abdomen.

In the late afternoon, the nurse arrived offering me a cup of tea which I gladly accepted. While enjoying my tea, I noticed that my heart had started to race and there was an intense feeling of warmth waving up from my feet towards my chest. I wondered what was happening and, on touching my chest, I noticed my skin had become wet. I wondered if I was having a hot flush. At that moment a nurse arrived and I asked her if that was what was happening and having been through the menopause herself, she confirmed that it sounded very much like it. I was very surprised that they had started so soon after surgery, but otherwise they were harmless and didn't bother me. Considering that I was now a menopausal woman at the young age of 35, however, did feel a little bizarre.

That night I slept well, but awoke around 4 am and, remembering that I had had surgery the day before, I struggled to get back off to sleep. As soon as visiting hours arrived, so too did my husband; I was delighted to see him. Mr Drake arrived on his morning rounds and explained that, all being well, I would be able to go home. However, I didn't feel at all ready to do so. I was still feeling frightened about so many things and, in particular, the fear of developing complications (even though this was probably unlikely at this point). Furthermore, I felt that I needed the space to rest, not only physically but emotionally as well, and I feared that this would be nearly impossible with two young children at home. He understood and said it would be fine to stay in another night, if that was best for me.

As the day progressed, I felt a little more comfortable and confident enough to try walking around, which the nurse said would help to alleviate the discomfort in my abdomen. I carefully sat on the edge of the bed and, pausing for a brief moment, I slowly stood up. To my surprise, I felt a little weak and wobbly on my feet but, with my husband on one side of me and the nurse on the other, I was confident enough to take a few steps. Very quickly, I felt steady enough to walk towards the chair, to try sitting for a while. However, sitting seemed to worsen the discomfort of my distended abdomen, and it was then that I noticed just how swollen it was. I sat there for as long as I possibly could, but it was too uncomfortable. I couldn't stay there any longer and headed back to my bed.

I didn't experience any further hot flushes during the day, but I had a couple through the following night which woke me up for a few minutes each time. However, even with these night sweats, I enjoyed a much deeper and more restful night's sleep and felt much more ready to go home the next day.

In the morning, the nurse removed the dressings covering each incision to check for any sign of infection and to apply new ones ready for me to go home. I was intrigued to see the incisions and, when I did, I was surprised at how small and neat they were. Thankfully, there were no signs of infection.

The nurse advised me to take things easy at home; to listen to my body and to rest when I felt the need. She explained that I might feel weak and tired for the next one to two weeks, but that this would eventually pass, and that I might experience shoulder pain, due to the gas which is put into the abdomen during surgery, but reassured me that it would resolve, along with the bloated abdomen, within a week or so. To ease any discomfort, she recommended taking pain medication, including paracetamol and ibuprofen, which I would be given just before discharge.

She advised against lying flat at night and recommended elevating my head on several pillows, with another under my knees, for comfort and also to decrease the risk of developing pain in my shoulder. She also recommended loose, comfortable clothing, to continue wearing my anti-DVT socks and to look out for any changes, such as oozing or redness/swelling around the incisions and a high temperature, which might suggest infection.

Moments later, my husband arrived with our children who were very excited to see me; I felt emotional seeing them again and was desperate to give them a kiss and cuddle. With the excitement of it all, I quickly realised how tired I was, still recovering from surgery. Nonetheless, I was delighted at the thought of being able to recover in the comfort of my own home.

Feeling a mixture of relief that it was all over, coupled with a fear of what was to come, I couldn't help but cry as we drove away from the hospital. I also found myself feeling a sense of guilt, and sadness, that I had been able to spare myself the possibility of ovarian cancer while my mum hadn't been so lucky.

Settling back in at home, I enjoyed being with my family and was pleased to have the first surgery out of the way. The following morning I had an appointment with my breast surgeon which, even despite my very recent surgery, I chose not to rearrange as I didn't want to delay any further the date for my mastectomy. I wanted the peace of mind, both from a cancer perspective and with regard to being menopausal without HRT.

My breast surgeon agreed that I should avoid starting HRT until after my mastectomy as it could increase the risk of breast cancer, but he reassured me that I wouldn't have to manage without it for long as he would most likely perform the operation within the next two to three months. In the meantime, he examined my breasts and, once again, reassured me that he found nothing of concern. He also explained that, according to evidence, my risk of breast cancer had decreased by 50% now that my ovaries had been removed. Over the next few days, I enjoyed the company of friends and appreciated life feeling as close to normal as possible. As the days passed, my physical discomfort slowly eased and the pain from the incisions all but disappeared, but I noticed that I hadn't opened my bowels since being in hospital. I wondered if perhaps this was because I hadn't been eating much and because I was less mobile than normal but, whatever the cause, I thought it would be fine. However, four days after my surgery, I realised that I was extremely constipated.

I sat on the toilet, on and off, for most of the day, but nothing was happening. I booked an emergency appointment with my family doctor who prescribed a mini-enema to use at home but, still, nothing happened. By the evening, I was growing increasingly more exhausted, and I even started to feel quite frightened by the whole ordeal. I called the hospital and Mr Drake requested that I come in for treatment, explaining that the significant constipation was most likely to have been caused by the morphine and, to a lesser degree, by the anaesthetic drug. However, he reassured me that he didn't anticipate any further problems once this was resolved and I had returned to eating normally.

Having to face returning to hospital, even just for an enema, was distressing. Arriving back in the surgical ward, one of the nurses who had looked after me during my stay showed me and my husband to a spare room and explained that a doctor would be in to see me shortly. Once the doctor had been in to confirm both that I needed an enema and that I wasn't allergic to any of the ingredients, the nurse arrived with the enema in hand. She inserted a large syringe full of liquid into my bottom and within seconds it was working; I knew I had to get to the toilet faster than ever. Fortunately, I made it in time and with what felt bizarrely similar to child-birth (albeit without any pain), out came the biggest stool I have ever seen in my life. No wonder I couldn't pass it naturally! I could hear my husband, who was sitting in the chair in the bedroom, in hysterics. Peering round the bathroom door, I too couldn't help but burst into laughter at what had just happened.

Now that that was out of the way, I was relieved to feel much more comfortable and, for the first time that day, I was able to sit down with ease. Almost immediately, I felt hungry and sharing this with my husband he, once again, fell about laughing in his chair. Moments later, the nurse came in to check on me and, trying my hardest to keep a straight face, I explained that it had resolved the issue. But, looking over at my husband, that was it, we both set each other off again. She smiled knowingly, probably having seen it many times before. She offered to fetch us a cup of tea which went down particularly well after the night's events. Close to midnight by now, we headed back home.

When I awoke the following morning, despite feeling much more comfortable, I didn't feel at all well; I was completely drained, and emotional, from the events of the day before. I felt scared of the effect that removing my ovaries would have on my future health, but I knew that there was no turning back now; my ovaries were gone. I felt a sense of grief at what might now be lost from my life for evermore; maybe my love life, maybe my overall health and sense of wellbeing. At this moment, I felt that going through all of this at the relatively young age of 35 was unfair. Only naturally, I felt a sense of anger towards life and what it had thrown my way.

Over the course of the next couple of days, and about a week after surgery, I continued to feel drained. I noticed that my eyes started to feel unusually dry. I also experienced unusual pains in my head and, on one occasion, these pains were also accompanied by a very brief disturbance to my vision, along with an immediate sense of being even more drained of energy. I believe this was some form of migraine. I had not experienced anything of this nature prior to surgery and, therefore, it seemed logical to me to attribute it to the effects of low oestrogen (as migraine is associated with menopause) and perhaps also partly due to the intense stress of the last few days. However, I am pleased to say that these symptoms resolved quickly and I have not experienced anything of this nature since.

Within one to two weeks after surgery, I started to feel much more comfortable; my distended abdomen had mostly resolved and I began to feel stronger and less tired. To my surprise, I didn't tend to experience hot flushes during the daytime but, on the occasions that I did, they only seemed to occur in response to heightened emotions, such as stress or excitement.

I continued to have two to three night sweats every night, but this would only disturb my sleep for what seemed to be just a few minutes at a time. I would awake to my heart racing, a feeling of intense heat and wetness, particularly on my chest, but within a few seconds I was able to fall back to sleep, at least until the next one arrived. In the mornings, only naturally, I felt a little more tired than usual, but it was perfectly manageable. I was able to continue with the day-to-day demands of everyday life which was a blessing, given that my life was very demanding with a young family.

I also noticed during this period that I was having vivid (but not bad) dreams, which I had read could be a symptom of the menopause. This is not something that I had experienced prior to surgery and, again, it was clear to me that these were happening as a result of low oestrogen.

Overall, however, going through this surgery and the recovery period which followed was a breeze compared with what I had imagined. Personally, if I had to go through it again (which of course won't be necessary), I wouldn't be fearful in any way of the surgery, the recovery or the menopause itself. I felt, and have continued to feel ever since, remarkably untroubled by menopausal symptoms; if this was all that the menopause had to bring then it was fine by me. Above all, my biggest sense of relief was still feeling like my normal self and the same person I had always been.

A couple of weeks after my surgery, I went back for a follow-up appointment with Mr Drake to learn of the findings from my ovaries and fallopian tubes. I walked into his consulting room, nervous of what I might hear. Sensing my nerves, he immediately reassured me that the ovaries and tubes were entirely normal, with no sign of atypia or malignancy. It took me a moment for his words to fully sink in, but when they did, I felt emotions of relief and happiness that I would almost certainly not be diagnosed with, or die from, ovarian cancer during my lifetime; however, mixed with these emotions was a sense of sadness for my mum, and for all the other women for whom this hadn't been possible.

For what was the first time since my mum's illness, I was completely free of the worry of ovarian cancer. I felt a weight lift from my shoulders and I felt lighter, and freer, than I had for years – I realised at that moment that the worry of ovarian cancer had been with me ever since my mum's illness. I looked over at my husband who was also smiling; we momentarily held each other's gaze. I turned to Mr Drake and thanked him for everything and for most probably saving my life. He smiled and nodded, clearly very pleased for us both.

Moving on from the results, he raised the importance of having a bone density scan, as soon as possible, to check the current health of my bones and to act as a baseline for future scans to be compared with. I assured him that I would request this, as quickly as possible, via my family doctor. He explained that once my mastectomy was over and done with, he would prescribe Elleste Duet Conti, a combined HRT containing the maximum dose of oestrogen as, in his experience, patients had responded well to this therapy. He also reassured me, once again, that a lack of oestrogen in the short term would not pose a risk for osteoporosis.

He recommended removing my anti-DVT socks, which I did there and then, desperate to be free of them. Towards the end of the meeting, I wanted to know when it would be acceptable for my husband and I to make love again; he reassured me that it would be fine to do so whenever we felt ready. With this, I explained my concern over developing vaginal dryness, particularly so with not starting HRT until after my mastectomy, but, to my surprise, he didn't seem concerned that this would be a problem, even months down the line, without HRT. I was very surprised to hear this; vaginal dryness is something that I thought would be a certainty with the menopause. However, he explained that if this did become a problem at any point in the future, even after starting HRT, then a vaginal oestrogen cream could be prescribed to alleviate this.

A couple of days later, and just over a fortnight after my surgery, my husband and I enjoyed a romantic evening together. We took things gently for fear that it may be painful, but, to my surprise, there was no pain or discomfort and making love felt the same as it had done prior to my surgery. In fact, making love on this first occasion after surgery felt particularly special, after what we had both experienced together over the last couple of weeks. Furthermore, being able to make love free of the worry of contraception and pregnancy was also very liberating.

Within only a month after surgery, I felt fully recovered. Life quickly returned to normal and I continued to enjoy being free of the worry of ovarian cancer. Only naturally, I continued to fear what removing my ovaries might have done to my overall health, but what was done was done, and I began to feel more secure with the knowledge that I would deal with whatever arose, if and when it ever happened. The fear of having a mastectomy in the near future continued to hang over me, but at the same time

I felt pleased that the end would soon be in sight – I had come this far and I knew that I would get through the remaining part of the journey.

During this time, my husband expressed concern at how slim I had become, but I knew from past experience with my mum's illness that this was my body's response to extreme stress. Even so, I was still surprised to lose weight as I had feared the opposite would happen now that my ovaries had been removed. I continued to eat healthily, as I had always done, to support my body through this challenging time and, approximately four weeks after surgery, I felt ready to return to exercise – a sign which I knew meant that I had recovered and that my body was coping well with what it had endured.

It was a great feeling being able to enjoy once again the sense of wellbeing that exercise brings. However, I noticed that while I was still able to keep up pace and complete the exercise as normal, my endurance was less, making the exercise feel harder. This loss of endurance was most probably due to having low oestrogen and the fact that it can take a long time after surgery or illness to regain the last few percentage points of fitness and energy. This resolved slowly over the course of the first year and, thankfully, it is not something that I ever experienced during the demands of normal, everyday life.

Very quickly after my ovaries had been removed, I started to experience an unpleasant tingling sensation around my urethra, which came and went throughout the day. My gynaecologist explained that the urethra tends to develop this sensation after oophorectomy as, similar to the vagina, it is sensitive to the effects of decreased oestrogen. A couple of months after my surgery, I also developed a sensation of pressure in my bladder as though it was full, even though I knew it wasn't, along with a slightly discoloured vaginal discharge. I visited my family doctor, suspecting that I might have a urinary tract infection (UTI) but, to my surprise, my urine was clear. However, I couldn't shrug off the feeling that something was amiss. I went back to my family doctor and, this time, she recommended sending a vaginal swab off to the hospital; this revealed a heavy infection with *Streptococci Group A*. I was given a course of antibiotics, which cleared it. Given that I had not suffered any infections of this nature prior to removing my ovaries and, given that evidence suggests it is associated with oestrogen deficiency,[1] it is reasonable to assume that this infection occurred as a consequence of my operation.

Around this time, I also noticed that I had been feeling teary and my mood was lower than usual but, while this might partly be explained by the effects of the menopause, this period of time in my life was clearly not an easy one. Feeling that I was perhaps beginning to struggle with the symptoms of the menopause, and with the worry of breast cancer continuing to hang over me, I requested an appointment to see my breast surgeon to see if I could be given a firm date for surgery. I wanted my mastectomy over and done with so that I could start taking HRT to alleviate my symptoms and so that this whole journey could soon be completed.

In the light of my symptoms, Mr Tyler reassured me that he would perform the surgery imminently and he took this opportunity to explain what the breast reconstruction process would involve, using the most recently released bovine STRATTICE™.

While examining my breasts, we discussed which size implant would be the most suitable for my body. I explained that I was not at all concerned by what size they would be post-surgery; I was happy for him to use whichever size implant he felt would be best. He asked if I had ever seen, or held, an implant before – I hadn't, but I was intrigued to see what one would look and feel like. He fetched two different sized implants – one which would reconstruct me to my current breast size and the other which would be approximately a cup-size larger. He explained that he would have a better idea during the surgery itself which size would be best, once he could see how much skin there would be after all of the breast tissue had been removed. I was reassured by his expertise and trusted that he would make the best decision for me on the day.

Within a day or so, I received a date for my mastectomy to be performed in a month's time at Stoke Mandeville Hospital. I felt a mixture of emotions from relief at finally having a date booked, through to fear and dread of what was to come. But, at least now, I had something concrete to work towards and to prepare myself for. Once again, I felt empowered and back in control of my destiny. The heavy burden of future surgery that I had been carrying for months seemed to lift and, momentarily, I felt excited that the end of my journey was now truly in sight. But, at the same time, my anxiety levels soared to a whole new level. I dreaded the prospect of further surgery and, above all, of losing my natural breasts. I was overcome by intense feelings of grief and sadness. Tears started rolling down my cheeks and I noticed my arm had moved across the front of my chest, as though I was protecting my breasts from what was coming.

Just over a week before my surgery, I went back to the hospital for my pre-op assessment, which involved various tests, including an electrocardiogram (ECG) to check that my heart was fit for surgery. Following this, I had an appointment with Mr Tyler and his team of surgeons. There seemed to be a very serious atmosphere in the room that hadn't been there during previous appointments; this, along with my surgery being imminent, made it all feel very, very real.

Noticing that I was on the verge of tears, one of the doctors asked how I was feeling. Trying hard not to cry, especially in front of so many doctors, I explained to him that with it having been such a huge emotional rollercoaster over the last year or so, I was feeling that I had few reserves left to push through this final stage. He understood and sympathised how tough the last year must have been.

Examining me one more time before surgery, Mr Tyler

explained that he had made the decision to operate via the inframammary fold (IMF), so that I wouldn't be left with any visible scarring on my breasts. He reassured me that operating in this way was just as effective at removing the breast tissue as any other form of incision. However, he mentioned that, with this approach, there may be a slight increased risk of developing necrosis but that, being quite small-busted, a non-smoker and in good health overall, he was prepared to take that gamble. On the one hand, I was delighted by the possibility of having no visible scarring while, at the same time, being particularly frightened by the possibility of developing necrosis. I reassured myself that I was in excellent hands in his care and that he would only do what was best for me.

Initially after surgery, he said to expect my entire breasts and chest area to feel numb but that, gradually in time, some of the feeling would return. He explained, however, that the erotic sensation would most likely be lost. He also explained that, immediately after surgery, the nipples would be paralysed and would not respond to temperature or touch, although, in time as the nerves in the skin started to regrow, they would function again.

Visit to a breast reconstruction awareness (BRA) group

A couple of days later, and a little under a week before my surgery, I attended a breast reconstruction awareness (BRA) group at the John Radcliffe Hospital, which is a support group to help women through cancer-related breast reconstruction surgery. It was led by one of the plastic and reconstructive surgeons who talked through each of the different options for reconstruction and what to expect in and around the time of admission and after surgery. In the second part of the meeting, there was an opportunity to meet with women who had already undergone a breast mastectomy with reconstruction, either as a risk-reducing strategy or following cancer. This enabled me to see each of the different types of reconstruction, something that, so far, I hadn't had the opportunity to do; it was very important for me to see what I could expect my breast reconstruction to look like and I was very grateful for the opportunity.

One of the women, also a BRCA2 mutation carrier, had undergone a risk-reducing mastectomy with DIEP flap reconstruction. A nipple had been reconstructed by pinching together a small bit of skin which was later tattooed to re-create the colouring of the nipple-areola complex. Her breasts looked so good that had I seen them in a different setting, I never would have known that they had been reconstructed. It is incredible just how good breast reconstruction can be. What also struck me was how positive she was about what she had gone through; it showed me that life would one day return to normal.

One of the other women had undergone a nipple-sparing mastectomy with implant-based reconstruction and, as this was my choice, I was eager to speak with her, to hear her own experience and to take a closer look at her reconstruction. Her breasts also looked very good and, had this been in a different setting, I would have thought that she had undergone an augmentation procedure and never a mastectomy with reconstruction. She, too, was very positive about her experience and it was clear to me that she loved her breasts – and so much so that she continued to enjoy going topless on holidays. Her only sadness, and the only thing that reduced her to tears, she explained, was the loss of the erotic sensation, which I empathised with, knowing that imminently I, too, would experience this.

Attending this meeting was very helpful and informative. What really struck me meeting these women was their strength and their sense of pride with what they had come through. I was also nicely surprised by their apparent love for their reconstructed breasts. I made the decision that just as soon as I felt ready to,

I, too, would one day attend and show my reconstruction to help others in the same way.

While this evening was extremely helpful, and positive in many ways, I still couldn't escape the feeling of, ultimately, not wanting to lose my natural breasts. After arriving home and, despite it being late, I made a camomile tea to help relax me and to take some time to process the night's events. I needed some space and time alone to think things through. Despite taking this time, however, I struggled to sleep. My mind was going over and over the evening's meeting and my forthcoming surgery. I awoke in the early hours of the morning, feeling intensely alone, frightened and, for first time throughout this journey, angry. Very angry!

Flashing through my mind was everything that life had ever thrown at me. I felt anger that I had lost my mum, and at such a young age, and anger towards all of the major events that I had had to overcome. And, now I had to face losing my breasts and the unknown of how this would impact me mentally and emotionally. I was terrified that I would awake from surgery feeling mutilated or maybe even violated, but this was one fear, one emotion, that I hadn't been able to share with anyone.

I continued to feel very heavy-hearted the following morning, but seeing my son beam a beautiful smile towards me helped to lift my spirits. Later that day, we had his 4th birthday party. Despite the strain I was under, I wanted life to continue as normal for the children's sake and to celebrate his birthday as we had always done in previous years. It was a special day, after which I was able to focus my energy on preparing for surgery.

As the surgery date neared, I noticed that I had started to withdraw a little from external life; I just wanted to be close to my family and to be close to nature. I found walking in the woods particularly calming and soothing. However, with only a couple of days before surgery, I felt the need to speak with one of the breast care nurses, to talk through some of my fears and emotions. She reassured me that how I was feeling was entirely normal and that she would be available to talk again if ever I felt the need. Talking through my emotions with someone who I knew would understand helped a great deal.

Undergoing a nipple-sparing mastectomy

On the morning of my mastectomy operation, I awoke with a sense of dread, but, surprisingly, also a sense of excitement that the operation day was finally here and that it would soon all be over. However, even with the months of preparation, I still didn't feel emotionally ready to undergo this surgery; then again, I don't think I would ever have felt ready.

Arriving at the hospital, the sense of dread became stronger than ever and I considered, for a very brief moment, not going ahead. I wanted to go home and forget about it all but, at the same time, I knew this wouldn't have been sensible. Instead, I forced myself to go through the motions, step by step, one foot in front of the other.

Walking along the corridor towards the Day Procedures Unit, panic started to build inside me. 'Just maybe I won't get breast cancer. Maybe I will be okay. Maybe I don't have to do this?!' I blurted out to my husband. I considered running; running as fast as possible away from the hospital. I wondered if I would be able to out-run my husband if he tried to catch me – I probably could have done in the circumstances. But, all the while, there was this little voice of reason reminding me that my risk of breast cancer was staggeringly high – there is just no running away from those statistics. If I did leave, I knew that I would always live in fear and, worse still, I might actually develop breast cancer. I didn't want to live with the regret of being diagnosed with it when I could have had a mastectomy to prevent it. That was enough for me to continue on ahead.

Arriving at the theatre reception, I fumbled for my paperwork, my hands shaking with nerves. I was handed a theatre gown and shown to a small private room to get changed. My hands were trembling, making it difficult to remove my clothes, and I began to feel cold with nerves. Feeling intense grief at imminently losing my breasts, tears started to roll down my cheeks; I looked at them one last time in the mirror and, in my own way, I said goodbye to them. I held them, one last time, trying to capture the memory of their softness and warmth in my hands.

Suddenly, my attention was drawn to a knock on the door; it was the nurse asking if I was ready to go through to see the anaesthetist. He introduced himself and explained that he would be looking after me during surgery. He had worked as an anaesthetist for many years and reassured me that he didn't anticipate any kind of complications. Surgery would last about four hours and, once they'd sent me off to sleep, I would be given a 'chest-block', which he described as a regional anaesthetic to reduce pain following surgery.

I explained that I was worried about the feeling of an elephant being on my chest after surgery which I had been told is often experienced by women awaking from a mastectomy. 'There will be no animals allowed in the operating theatre!' he responded, in an attempt to calm my nerves. We couldn't help but laugh and this helped to diffuse some of the tension.

A few minutes later, Mr Tyler arrived with several other doctors who I realised would be involved during my operation. 'Are we ready?' he asked. 'Yes,' I responded confidently, although on the inside I didn't feel quite so ready. He asked me to sit on the edge of the bed so that he could use a marker pen to mark the area which would be operated on during surgery. I felt quite exposed in front of so many male doctors, and indeed Mr Tyler had mentioned that I might feel this way, but I understood that they were ultimately just doing their job.

Ready for surgery, my husband and I headed with the doctors along the corridor to the pre-op room. Arriving at the door, my husband was told that he couldn't go any further. We said our quick goodbyes and I, hesitantly, entered. I was immediately taken aback by the warmest of greetings, similar to what I had experienced during my first operation. I couldn't help but break out into a smile; I knew that they were trying to ease my anxiety and, again, it worked.

I had a strong sense of *déjà vu*; the pre-op room looked identical to that for the first surgery, which I found a little unnerving, but I reassured myself that I had done it once, I could do it again. More confidently this time, I removed my dressing gown and slippers and climbed onto the bed. Within only a matter of minutes it seemed, the anaesthetist gave me the pre-op medication, explaining that I would feel very drunk as he did so. By this point, I felt quite relaxed and, a few seconds later, I saw him administer the anaesthetic. It was all nearly over, I reassured myself. I shut my eyes and moments later, I was asleep.

Awaking in recovery, it did indeed feel like there was a small elephant sitting on my chest. However, given that I was able to take a deep breath with ease, I wasn't alarmed by this sensation. I felt quite tired, but otherwise apart from the discomfort in my chest, I wasn't in any pain and I actually felt surprisingly well. I noticed that I was now wearing a skin-coloured, surgical bra which must have been put on me towards the end of surgery. I also noticed that there were plastic tubes coming out from the sides of my chest, which were filled with watery-looking blood.

The anaesthetist came over and reassured me that the operation had gone very smoothly and that all was well. Within a short while, I was wheeled to the ward where my husband was waiting for me. I was pleased to see him and relieved that it was all over – no more surgery, all being well, I thought.

I had done it; I had now done everything in my power to prevent being diagnosed with breast and ovarian cancer during my lifetime. Even in amongst my fear, I felt a deep sense of pride at what I had achieved and for finding the bravery to undergo two life-changing operations. And, seeing how much my husband loved me and how proud he was of me gave me the strength and the conviction that I would get through my recovery.

My husband explained to me that Mr Tyler had already been to see him to reassure him that everything had gone smoothly and that he would expect me to feel very happy with the reconstruction. Mr Tyler had explained also that he had needed to use the larger of the two implants, which he had placed under the chest muscles, as there had been more skin than he had anticipated; skin which was present as a result of the rapid increase in breast size during pregnancy and, furthermore, during breastfeeding. I was very relieved to hear that things had gone as well as they had.

A short while later, a nurse arrived to see how I was feeling and to explain that there was a patient-controlled analgesia (PCA), containing morphine, at the side of my bed, which I could press for pain relief as and when I needed to. She also gave me various pain medications, including paracetamol, ibuprofen and codeine and a laxative to try to prevent a recurrence of the constipation I had experienced after my first surgery. I could see also that I was being given intravenous antibiotics through the cannula in the back of my hand to reduce the risk of infection.

She explained the need to keep myself upright at a 45-degree angle for the next few days to help reduce the swelling and bruising across my chest. I asked if it would be possible to have some extra padding to cover my chest as this had been one of the recommendations given at the BRA group that I had attended. It had been explained that keeping the chest very warm after surgery helps to keep the blood flow open to the skin which, in turn, helps to prevent necrosis. The nurse came back with a large, square-shaped piece of bandage which looked like a large padded wad of cotton wool. It did the job perfectly well, but I was almost unbearably hot with it on.

Being late and past visiting hours, my husband was encouraged to leave to allow me to get some rest. Lying there, on raised pillows, I noticed that I now had more of a cleavage than prior to surgery. I also took a closer look at the surgical drains (two coming out just to the side of each breast) which were collecting the excess fluid accumulating in the area where the mastectomy had been performed. I wasn't fazed by the site of these; in fact, loving anything medical, I was actually quite intrigued by them.

Mr Tyler arrived with one of his doctors to check that my recovery was running smoothly. Unfastening the grippers down the front of my surgical bra, he inspected my breasts very thoroughly. My entire chest felt very numb; I couldn't feel the doctor's fingers touching my skin, but I could feel a sense of pressure which was a bizarre and unpleasant sensation. To my relief, he was happy that there were no signs of necrosis or anything of any concern at all. Mr Tyler's team continued to monitor me carefully throughout the night which gave me reassurance and helped to ease my anxieties.

Despite being exhausted, I only managed to sleep a few minutes here or there, partly due to the noise levels on the ward, but mostly because I was petrified of developing complications. In the middle of the night, during one of the nurse's rounds, I told her that I was feeling panicky; it almost felt as if I was having a fight-or-flight response. She reassured me that she saw this response often in people who had just undergone major surgery and that it would pass.

By the morning I was very tired after little sleep and, now that the chest-block had worn off, I also felt extremely sore and uncomfortable. The nurse arrived to take away my PCA, to my complete shock and horror. I was in a lot of discomfort and the only thing really bringing any form of relief was the morphine – the thought of managing without it was alarming to say the least. Wanting to cling on to it and refusing to give it back, I explained that I didn't feel that paracetamol, ibuprofen and codeine alone would be sufficient. She explained, because morphine is highly addictive, there is a need to minimise its usage and she tried to reassure me that, in her experience, patients tend to manage well without it. With that, my morphine was gone.

As soon as visiting hours arrived, so too did my husband. Laying eyes on him, I felt immediately brighter and more positive. Feeling safe with him by my side, I was able to fall asleep for a couple of hours and felt much better for the rest. Shortly after waking up, the nurse suggested that I try to walk to the toilet, to start becoming more mobile. I found it very difficult to reposition myself as using my hands to push down on the bed, or putting any kind of strain on my chest was out of the question. Slowly, but surely, I worked my way to the edge of the bed and, to my surprise, I felt steady on my feet and capable of walking alone.

Coming back from the toilet, the enormity of what I had been through seemed to hit me. Again, I felt panicked and wanted to run, but I'm sure that I wouldn't have got very far with four drains trailing behind me and what a sight that would have been! How I felt at this moment was probably the worst of my entire journey. It was as though I had lost all my composure and it took every bit of my strength to remain calm and controlled.

Walking back to the chair next to the bed, the nurse arrived to check my vital signs. I saw that my blood pressure was sky high at 125/178 mm Hg, far higher than my normal level. However, she didn't seem at all concerned and explained that it was most likely because I had just walked around for the first time. Personally, I was terrified that this was a sign that something was going wrong in my recovery, only adding further to my already panicked state. Again, the nurse reassured me that I was doing very well post-operatively and that everything was fine. With this, and with a reassuring cuddle from my husband, I gradually managed to calm down.

Later that night, feeling physically and emotionally drained, I started to cry at the thought of how much I missed my children. The nurse arrived at that moment and noticed that I was crying. She was a wonderful support and shared with me her admiration for how well I had coped with the recovery and how strong I had been facing a mastectomy at such a young age. On top of this, she said how well I looked for someone who had just gone through a mastectomy. Her kind words gave me a little boost and a confidence that, despite my emotional wobble, I was actually doing very well in my recovery.

I didn't manage to get any sleep at all that night with the noise levels on the ward, and I felt probably the most exhausted I had ever been in my entire life. I was glad when morning finally arrived, knowing that it wouldn't be long before I would be able to go home. After breakfast, the nurse arrived to prepare me for discharge. She showed me how to empty my drains and recommended doing so as and when the bags became full. She then removed one of the two drains from either side of my breast and put on fresh drainage bags at the ends of the remaining two. The sensation of the drains being removed was very unpleasant and unlike any sensation I had felt before but, thankfully, it was over and done with within a matter of seconds and, once they were gone, I immediately felt more comfortable. Looking at my chest, I could see that bruising was starting to develop in patches across my breasts and there was also visible swelling but, otherwise, they looked good and I was pleased that there was no visible scarring.

The nurse removed the cannula through which I had been receiving intravenous antibiotics, and briefed me on my discharge meds and when to take them, including ibuprofen and paracetamol for pain relief, lactulose to prevent constipation and a two-week course of antibiotics to reduce the risk of infection. I was advised not to lift anything heavy, and certainly nothing heavier than a bag of sugar, for six weeks, until fully recovered. She explained that I would be seen by Mr Tyler twice a week, and that the two drains would remain for the next 10 or so days. I thanked the nurse for looking after me and, within moments, the wheelchair arrived to take me to the car. To try to lift my spirits, and whenever it was safe to do so, my husband enjoyed pushing me along speedily back to the car. I couldn't stop myself from laughing, but it was uncomfortable. Nonetheless, how lovely it was to laugh again after the events of the last two days.

Arriving back home, I continued to be in a lot of discomfort and felt completely drained of all energy. My children ran to the front door, delighted to see me, as I was them. Hearing their little voices and seeing their faces made me feel emotional. I wanted to give them a big cuddle, but it was nearly impossible with the drains in the way. My chest felt very vulnerable and I didn't feel at ease with anyone being close to it.

Sitting down in the lounge where I would be most comfortable, I tried my hardest to appear happy and upbeat, as I would normally be, but this was very difficult given how much discomfort I was in. I noticed my children's concern for me and, in particular, I noticed that my son was a little frightened by my drains which, despite my best efforts to hide them, were still slightly visible. I reassured them both that they were helping mummy get better and that everything was okay. 'Mummy, do you have pretend boobies now?' he asked. 'Yes, I do, darling!' I responded trying to sound cheerful. 'Can I see them, Mummy?' he asked. We all broke into laughter.

Being back in the comfort of my own home was heavenly and I managed to have a much better night's sleep, albeit I still found it uncomfortable to sleep at a 45-degree angle. The following morning, and now three days after surgery, I felt a little less tired, but I continued to be in a great deal of discomfort. I simply couldn't tolerate the pain anymore – managing on paracetamol and ibuprofen, for me personally, was not enough. I asked my husband to 'phone the hospital and they requested that I return for a prescription of codeine, an opiate analgesic, which I was advised to take along with the other medications. At the hospital, the doctor gave me the prescription and also took the opportunity to examine me. He was very pleased and surprised at how well I was recovering, commenting that I was very mobile, and that the incisions were healing particularly quickly and neatly. Thankfully, the codeine helped to take the edge off the pain, reducing the discomfort to a more manageable level.

The following day, even though I had been advised not to shower while the drains were in place, I found that having a shallow bath helped me to stay fresh and to feel in good spirits. I was then able to carefully lean over the edge of the bath tub just long enough to have my husband wash my hair. Looking in the mirror after my bath, I could see that there was now extensive yellow bruising across most of my breasts, as well as patches of purple and black on and around my nipples. Seeing this level of bruising was quite shocking and also a little frightening; my poor breasts had really been through it. Gently touching them to see how they felt, I now understood what Mr Tyler had meant when he explained that they would feel very firm, with little, if any, movement. However, even though they didn't feel like natural breasts, their shape and form were beautiful and I knew that once the bruising had gone, they would look incredible. I got dressed into some comfortable clothes and enjoyed putting some earrings in for the first time – just something as simple as that helped me to feel brighter and more human again.

Later that morning, I had my first follow-up appointment with Mr Tyler. Arriving at the hospital a little early, I grabbed a quick coffee from the cafe. Sitting in one of the chairs was an expectant mother who was in the early stages of labour. A beautiful sight, I thought, but almost immediately I was overcome by sadness and grief and, with this, I began to cry. Not so long ago, I was pregnant and going through labour and now here I was having had both ovaries removed and in a lot of discomfort recovering from a mastectomy. How quickly life can change.

Arriving in the busy waiting area, and feeling so physically and emotionally drained, I started to cry, once again, but this time I knew the tears wouldn't stop so quickly. I was exhausted, which was only adding to my emotional state, and I had had enough of the pain and discomfort – I desperately wanted my recovery and this period of my life over and done with.

A few minutes later, I heard Mr Tyler call my name. I walked through with tears still streaming down my face – I couldn't even bring myself to wipe them away. Mr Tyler showed great compassion and reassured me that I was recovering about as well as I could possibly be. He explained that the bruising was already beginning to fade and from now on, he said, it would fade from yellow to green and, finally, through to a musty brown colour. I was also pleased to hear that I could now lie down flat in bed, as trying to sleep at the 45-degree angle made it nearly impossible to get a good night's rest. I noticed also that there was a thumb-size dip in the left side of my left breast, as well as a small dip just beneath my right nipple, but Mr Tyler reassured me that given time these would disappear (and they did within a couple of months). He explained that they had struggled in surgery to get the skin to sit properly over the left implant and, therefore, they needed to do some specialist plastics work to resolve this.

After a very emotional morning, I started to feel better as the day progressed, helped by the fact that my pain levels were beginning to improve. That night, I tried to lie flat, as Mr Tyler had suggested, but I simply wasn't able to do so as it seemed to pull too much on my chest area, making it feel as if it would split open. Once again, my husband set my pillows up for me to sleep at a 45-degree angle.

The following day, and now five days after surgery, I continued to feel less emotional and, with this, I started to have the space for the positive emotions to begin to surface. I felt a deep sense of pride for finding the strength and the bravery necessary to go ahead with the surgery – it was 100% the right choice for me. I could now enjoy the tremendous relief that it was all over and done with. No more living in fear of breast cancer.

The following morning, and for the first time since my surgery,

I felt strong enough to have a walk around my local town centre and to go out for some lunch. Getting out and about, enjoying some fresh air and a taste of normality, was fantastic and it really lifted my spirits. Walking through town, I was surprised to notice that my breasts no longer bounced as my natural breasts used to.

Exactly a week after my mastectomy, I noticed a dramatic improvement; I now felt much more comfortable and, having slept much better, I also felt less tired. Looking at my breasts, I noticed that a black scab was starting to form over both nipples, particularly so on my left nipple. I was due to see Mr Tyler for a second follow-up appointment and, bringing this to his attention, he explained that these scabs were as a result of a minor level of necrosis. Hearing any mention of the word necrosis filled me with dread, but he reassured me that this was to be expected given how every effort had been made to remove as much breast tissue from behind the nipple as possible. He explained that the scab had formed because the blood flow to the nipple had not been adequate to support the tissue. However, new blood vessels would now be being formed to improve the blood flow and eventually the scabs would fall off revealing healthy, normal-coloured skin underneath.

I also mentioned that my reconstructed breasts tended to feel very cold, but that they fluctuated between feeling cold through to very warm. Bizarrely, sometimes one felt hot and the other cold. The reason for this, he explained, is because the implants tended to be a little cooler than the rest of the body as they were filled with silicone and sat outside the chest cavity, just beneath the skin. They themselves did not have a blood supply, but they were able to heat up and retain this heat, in which case they would feel warm, or they could lose this heat and, hence, feel cold.

He continued to be very happy with my recovery, and I was delighted to hear him describe my new breasts as 'perfect'. I agreed; they did look perfect. I felt very lucky to have had such a talented surgeon and I thanked him for what he had done for me. With my drains now collecting less and less fluid as the days passed, he felt confident that the last two drains would be removed during my next follow-up appointment, in only a few days' time. My left drain was becoming increasingly uncomfortable and, in fact, my only remaining discomfort seemed to be coming from them.

By nine days post-surgery, I didn't feel that I needed quite as much pain relief. Only occasionally did I feel any discomfort, but this resolved quickly with simple paracetamol and ibuprofen. I was now able to get myself in and out of the bath with ease and to wash my own hair by kneeling in the bath water, and carefully lifting my hands just enough to be able to reach my head. I continued to need help getting dressed, but I was getting there, slowly but surely.

Just as Mr Tyler had anticipated, my drains were removed during my next follow-up appointment, 11 days post-surgery. This time, they were a little more difficult to remove as my body had begun to heal around them. I experienced a hot, burning and a strong tugging sensation but, within a matter of seconds, it was all over and done with. Immediately, I felt a physical sense of relief from being free of the drains. Gone was my remaining discomfort – I lay there for a moment enjoying the feeling of being totally comfortable for the first time since surgery.

Whilst lying on the bed, I mentioned that I had recently been able to feel one or two tiny, circular bumps just sitting under the skin of my breasts. He explained that these were some of the internal stitches and that they would slowly dissolve over a period of many months, which they did. Mr Tyler advised that he would be happy for me to wear ordinary bras from now on, but he recommended avoiding underwired bras until at least six weeks post-surgery. I was advised to continue taking my antibiotics for a further 48 hours after the drain removal, and the pain medication as and when needed.

Now that the drains had been removed, not only did I find it easier to wash (and being able to shower again felt heavenly!), but I also found it much easier to dress myself. I enjoyed the feeling of being capable again and not reliant on others and this helped to boost me emotionally. Both my husband and I were pleasantly surprised that I was beginning to regain my independence.

Exactly two weeks post-surgery, I felt much better and any remaining discomfort was confined to first thing in the morning and was quickly relieved with the painkillers. Even though my breasts still looked sore with the bruising, they now looked worse than they felt. The swelling was passing and I could see clearly how my new breasts would soon appear. Most importantly, I was very happy with them; they looked amazing and I didn't feel in any way less of a woman or less attractive. I am also pleased to say that the surgery did not leave me feeling mutilated or violated, as I had feared. Psychologically, I felt very strong and confident that I would continue on with the positive self-image that I had enjoyed before my surgeries. Being confident of this was a deeply satisfying emotion to feel at a time which had for many months been filled with great fear and uncertainty.

When I returned to hospital for my two-week follow-up appointment, I was pleasantly surprised to hear the doctor describe my breasts as looking very nice. Hearing this from another man besides my husband, albeit a doctor, was lovely. Moments later, Mr Tyler arrived, accompanied by a trainee doctor and several other doctors whom I had met previously. With my permission, he explained to the trainee doctor the type of surgery that I had undergone and, as he did so, he was clearly delighted with the quality of his work. Once he was happy that everything was fine, I dressed and returned to the seat next to my husband. Unbeknownst to me, while I was getting dressed, Mr Tyler had briefly left the room to see if they had received the pathology back from my mastectomy. Walking back into the room, I heard the words, 'We've got your results and there was no sign of any atypia, DCIS or malignancy'. It suddenly hit me what was happening – these were my results and I was being given the all clear! There was no evidence of anything worrying at all – no abnormal-looking cells, no DCIS, no cancer. Time slowed down, everything started to feel surreal and almost dream-like. 'I'm all clear?' I asked, surprised to be learning of my results today. 'Yes, you are all clear.'

I felt lost for words. Immediately, the events of the last year or so flashed through my mind – from finding out that I carried a BRCA2 gene mutation, through the removal of my ovaries, having recently gone through a mastectomy and now being given the all clear. I had done it and I couldn't possibly have done more. This truly represented the end of my personal BRCA journey.

I felt a huge rush of emotion spread from my solar plexus throughout my whole body. I started to cry tears of relief and joy. I looked towards my husband who was smiling through his own tears. He pulled me gently toward him, wiping away my tears as he did so. With the good news sinking in more and more, I began to smile and, so much so, that I couldn't stop smiling. I looked up toward the many doctors standing around the room and I was pleasantly surprised to see that they, too, were all beaming. How lovely, I thought. They were clearly genuinely happy for me and I considered how moments like this must be among some of their most rewarding in their careers as doctors.

I left the hospital feeling elated and continued smiling the whole journey home. I reflected on the year that had passed – what a year that had been! I felt as if I had been dragged through the proverbial hedge a hundred times over but, nevertheless, I had got through it and it had all been worth it to be free of the worry of developing breast and ovarian cancer. Arriving home, I was eager to share our fantastic news with our children. Despite them being unaware of any pending results, I wanted them to know that everything was well and that all the operations were now finished. My daughter excitedly flung her arms around me, squeezing me tighter than she had ever done before. 'I really love you, Mummy!' she exclaimed. At the same time, my son also cheered and flung his arms around me. This was a beautiful moment for our family and I could now look forward to enjoying the year ahead, as well as many more happy years in the future.

Climbing into bed that night, still elated from the day's events, I took my first HRT pill. To my surprise I was able to sleep the whole night through without being awoken by any night sweats. I felt brilliant the next morning, amazed that I had slept so well. From that day on, I have never again experienced any hot flushes or night sweats and, within a day or so of starting the HRT, I also noticed that normal vaginal lubrication had returned.

By three weeks post-surgery, I was able to drive again although, initially, turning the wheel, which uses the chest muscles more than you'd imagine, felt uncomfortable. Nonetheless, getting my freedom back was a great feeling. I was also now able to lie flat on my back which made sleeping a whole lot easier. I disliked the feeling of lying on my side for some time after surgery, as resting on the side of the implant felt very strange and uncomfortable but, within a short period of time, this became easier. Furthermore, moving my arms became easier and less painful, although I continued to find it a little awkward doing simple things, such as putting a coat on, opening a car door, chopping or mashing a potato, or opening bottles, as these tasks seemed to put too much pressure on my chest. At times, when I might have overdone things a little, I noticed that my breasts would become slightly swollen, reminding me that I still needed to take things easy.

Often throughout my recovery, I would also experience an unpleasant pricking pain in my breasts which I can only describe as feeling similar to being stung by nettles. On a couple of occasions, I had an unbearable itching in them which I either felt unable to scratch because my skin felt sore to touch or, if I tried to scratch it, it was not relieved anyway. Unlike normal itching, it was also difficult to figure out exactly where the itch was coming from, which didn't help matters. Such symptoms of numbness, shooting or pricking pain, or unbearable itching are all part of the post-mastectomy pain syndrome (PMPS), which is thought to be linked to damage done to the nerves in the armpit and chest during surgery, although the exact causes are unknown.

A little over three weeks post-surgery, the small scab on my right nipple had fallen off, revealing healthy, normal-coloured skin beneath, whereas the scab on my left nipple was still hanging on by a small thread. Just behind this remaining scab, I noticed that white goo had formed. My immediate fear was that an infection had developed, but I reassured myself that this was unlikely with there being no signs of redness around the area, pain or temperature. I 'phoned the hospital and spoke with one of Mr Tyler's team and he was happy enough that there wasn't an infection, but suggested that I go to the hospital the following morning to get it seen by one of the doctors. To my relief, the following morning, all was well and the doctor removed the scab, explaining that, with the scab being mostly detached, it was the perfect breeding ground for bugs.

By four to five weeks post-surgery, all of my bruising had gone and my skin had returned to its normal colour. Now that my breasts were free of any swelling, bruising or scabs, it was possible to see how lovely my reconstructed breasts were. I was delighted with the results, they looked incredible. If I were to draw the most perfect looking breasts for my body, it would be the ones which Mr Tyler had constructed for me. Returning for a further follow-up, exactly one month after surgery, Mr Tyler confirmed that any swelling had resolved and my breasts had now settled into their final shape and size. All being well, he wouldn't need to see me again for six months.

A week later, and now six weeks post-surgery, I enjoyed being able to return to exercise, once again. Initially, I only felt comfortable starting with gentler forms, such as walking, cycling and yoga-pilates but, nonetheless, simply being able to exercise again felt amazing. To my surprise, I was able to exercise as well as I had done prior to surgery and I didn't experience any difficulty with rotational movements of either arm. However, lying flat on the floor and laying my left arm flat above my head felt as if the underside of my breast was about to split open. Fearing something was wrong, I booked an emergency appointment with Mr Tyler, but, to my relief, everything was okay. This sensation, he explained, was being caused by tightness in the lower part of the *pectoralis major* muscle – a thick, fan-shaped muscle situated in the chest – which is cut through close to the ribs and lifted up for the implant to be placed underneath. He advised that given time, this should resolve by itself, which I am pleased it mostly has. Only occasionally do I notice a slight tightness in this area at the start of exercise but, once I have warmed up, this sensation typically disappears.

To celebrate the end of my surgeries, we booked a family holiday to Lanzarote – never before had we deserved a holiday more than now. With this just round the corner, I had a good excuse to go shopping, both for some new holiday clothes and to treat myself to some new lingerie. I had been looking forward to this moment, which for me represented the end of my journey, for a long time. Being measured by a corsetière, I was now a 32D, one cup size larger than my natural breasts. I enjoyed trying on a whole variety of beautiful bra and knickers sets, including underwired bras, and I was pleased that the bras not only fitted perfectly, but they also felt entirely comfortable. One thing I have found is that bras with anything more than a little bit of padding, or bras which are designed to enhance the cleavage, are no longer comfortable. However, due to the reconstruction with implants, these bras are no longer needed as I have a lovely cleavage without them. Furthermore, what is also quite nice is to have the option of not wearing any bra at all, particularly so with dresses which are best worn without strap lines being visible.

Flying away on holiday, I felt that these operations were now a closed chapter of my life. However, I was aware that, emotionally, I needed a little bit of breathing space to recuperate and to come to terms with everything that I had endured over the last year or so. But, I knew that time would be a great healer and that eventually these feelings would fade.

Shortly after returning from our family holiday, and only as little as nine weeks after my surgery, I felt ready to return to the BRA group at John Radcliffe Hospital to show my breast reconstruction, in the hope of helping others. It was a deeply satisfying emotion to feel that I was giving something back to the group that had helped me. However, perhaps the nicest feeling of all was the realisation of just how quickly I felt back to being my normal self after surgery.

21.
Effect on my body image, identity and sexual functioning

In this chapter I share with you, openly and honestly, the effect that undergoing a risk-reducing BSO and mastectomy has had on my body image, identity and sexual functioning. I endeavour, wherever possible, to describe the effects of each surgery separately; however, as you will see, some of the effects are the result of a combination of both surgeries. It is important to note that what follows is *my* own experience, which may or may not be the experience of other women who undergo these procedures.

As far as having removed my ovaries is concerned, I am pleased to say that this surgery has not affected my body image or identity in any way. I feel that this is partly because these organs were internal to my body and, therefore, with nothing having changed on the outside, there has been no effect on my body image. Furthermore, because I feel very womanly for having borne two children, and because I had the certainty that my family was complete, removing my ovaries and, consequently, being sterile did not cause me any distress or upset. Only naturally, however, I have on a couple of occasions had brief moments of sadness, such as seeing a pregnant woman or a newborn baby, but I feel that this isn't too dissimilar to the emotions that many women feel when they are aware that they will have no further children, whether sterile or not.

Since having my ovaries removed, words cannot express just how happy and relieved I am to no longer suffer from pre-menstrual syndrome (PMS). Thankfully now, I no longer have to endure teary times around ovulation or the mood swings immediately before starting my period. The removal of my ovaries has, paradoxically, had a positive effect on my (and my husband's!) quality of life.

With regard to the surgically induced menopause, compared with the long list of frightening possibilities, mine was a walk in the park. To my surprise, it was limited to hot flushes, night sweats and vaginal dryness. I noticed that I was having more down days, which I would only experience very rarely before undergoing surgery, but my feeling is that this was a reflection of how much strain I was under, rather than solely of low oestrogen. On the whole, I felt remarkably unaffected by menopausal symptoms and, for this reason, it is not something that I would now fear in any way whatsoever – I wish I had known before my surgeries just how easy it would be for me.

The night sweats and hot flushes resolved immediately after starting HRT, and the vaginal dryness improved greatly. Despite my concerns over gaining weight as a result of the menopause, I needn't have worried about this either. I continue to be very slim and to enjoy an athletic body shape. In my experience of taking HRT, I found that it initially increased my appetite, but, within a few months or so, this levelled off, just as my gynaecologist had suggested that it would. In my mind, the benefit of taking the HRT far outweighs the potential for weight gain and I will happily continue taking it until the natural age that menopause would have occurred, to derive all of the oestrogen-related benefits. With regard to the condition of my skin, hair and nails, removing my ovaries has not negatively affected them in any way.

With regard to the effect of these surgeries on my love life, very soon after undergoing surgery to remove my ovaries I noticed a considerable loss of sensation during intercourse which, only naturally, affected my enjoyment of sex and my ability to achieve orgasm. I was aware of the possibility of a loss of sensation having seen the medical literature, with roughly half of women reporting decreased sexual satisfaction after oophorectomy, but I tried my best to keep an open mind as to what my own experience would be, as everyone is different. This loss of sensation was not something that was present prior to the removal of my ovaries and, therefore, it is fair to assume that it was a consequence of my surgery, in some way. On a positive note, however, the sensation from clitoral stimulation was unaffected and my ability to achieve orgasm through this form of stimulation was also unaffected. Despite my concern over the loss of sensation, I was thankful that I was still able to orgasm, and that the quality and intensity of this were unchanged.

In addition to this, during the three-month period between removing my ovaries and undergoing a mastectomy (during which time I was not taking HRT), I experienced vaginal dryness. This sometimes resulted in sex feeling a little painful, along with a sensation that I can only describe as 'skin on skin'. As a result, making love didn't feel as pleasurable or as enjoyable as it had been prior to surgery. However, to my surprise, this vaginal dryness was not as bad, or as problematic, as I had expected it to be. There was still natural lubrication present, it wasn't 'dry' as the name suggests (and there was no cracking or bleeding), but the moisture was less at the entrance to the vagina, making intercourse a little more difficult and, at times, slightly uncomfortable. Thankfully, this discomfort would pass within a minute or two. To my surprise, also, after we started to make love, more lubrication would occur naturally, helping to make things flow better, but sometimes it wasn't quite enough for things to flow smoothly. On a couple of occasions, we tried using lubrication which eased the problem, but the lubrication itself tended to cause stinging and, therefore, this wasn't really an option for me. Thankfully, once I was able to start HRT, this vaginal dryness improved greatly but, even so, at times it would feel that there wasn't quite enough lubrication for things to flow well.

Whilst we continued to make love throughout these challenges, the loss of sensation continued to be apparent and gradually, over time, it was this that started to have a negative impact on our love life. Questioning whether there would be a loss of sensation each time we made love only compounded the problem further, making it increasingly difficult for me, and for my husband, to switch off and enjoy the moment. Thankfully, my husband was amazing throughout and supported me every step of the way, reassuring me that we would work through it together, which we did.

At one of my lowest points, approximately nine months after having had my ovaries removed (and six months after my mastectomy), I started to feel anxious about making love for fear that it wouldn't be pleasurable and that, ultimately, the whole experience would be disappointing. I began to lose my confidence and that was really tough. Going through these kinds of emotions was alien to me; I had always enjoyed a healthy and satisfying love life. Perhaps one of the worst emotions was that I began to feel that I was different from other women because I no longer felt able to enjoy the sex life that I had been used to and which, only naturally, I imagined other women being able to enjoy. I didn't feel less of a woman feeling this way, but it was still a very unpleasant emotion to live through.

There was even a brief period of time when I felt that I had reached the end of my love life, forcing me to question whether my life could feel happy and complete without sex. But I didn't want this to be my reality; I wanted my love life to continue. Nonetheless, always looking for the positives in any situation, I reminded myself that even if this journey had been at the expense of my love life, at least I was alive and well. If I had kept my ovaries intact, and if I had followed the same fate as my mum and died of ovarian cancer, that too would have been the end of my love life!

Feeling that I was beginning to struggle with the vaginal dryness and a loss of sensation negatively impacting my enjoyment of sex, I booked an appointment with my family doctor. She felt it best to write to my consultant gynaecologist for advice on how to manage these symptoms. Mr Drake responded swiftly, recommending a topical vaginal oestrogen cream which could be directly inserted into the vagina to help relieve the remaining dryness. My family doctor then prescribed a cream called Ovestin, which I have continued to use twice weekly ever since. This cream has, in addition to the HRT, helped to further improve levels of vaginal moisture which, in turn, has helped to make sex more comfortable and, thus, more pleasurable. In addition to this, since using this cream on a regular basis, I have not developed any further vaginal or urinary tract infections and the prickly sensation around my urethra has almost entirely disappeared.

Things were on the up and, gradually over time, I regained my confidence and enjoyment of sex. Making love started to flow better, the sensation improved slightly (although it was still less than before surgery) and, with everything working better, my love life returned very closely to what it had been prior to undergoing risk-reducing surgery. The feeling of getting through the challenges and getting my love life back was one of the best feelings in the world. Overcoming these difficulties also made me appreciate being able to make love whereas, before my operations, this was perhaps something that I took for granted.

Initially, I had felt that the loss of sensation was occurring solely as a result of the physical effect that removing my ovaries was having on my body, but, gradually over a period of a year and a half following surgery, I began to realise that there was more to it than this. There would be times, for example, when the sensation was decreased, but then there would be other times where the sensation was good, such as when I was feeling particularly romantic, or after sharing a glass of wine together, which inevitably would have helped me to feel more relaxed.

If this loss of sensation had been solely caused by the loss of my ovaries, I would have expected it to be constant and not to vary over time. I came to the conclusion, therefore, that while the loss of my ovaries and the effect of low oestrogen and/or low testosterone might be partly responsible, there must have also been some kind of underlying emotional or psychological cause. I wondered if perhaps fearing that my love life would be negatively affected by removing my ovaries and worrying about this possibility had, on some level, caused exactly that to happen. The truth is I don't really know for sure. I don't think it will ever be possible to be certain of the cause but, what is certain is that the body's biggest sex organ is, in fact, the brain and what's going on in your head has an enormous influence on your pleasure and satisfaction.

Furthermore, I am confident that a degree of this loss of sensation during love making is attributable to the loss of the erotic sensation in my nipples after mastectomy. With this, I initially found it harder to become aroused and, for a while at least, this affected my ability to orgasm during intercourse. Eventually, after exploring other ways of helping me to become aroused, this has improved matters and my ability to orgasm has returned to that prior to surgery.

As far as my libido is concerned, I feel that there may have been a slight drop, but it is so slight that it is practically unremarkable. I continue to have a healthy desire for sex. One thing that I have noticed in this regard is that I no longer experience the 'must have it now' desire that I would often feel at the lead-up to ovulation or just prior to starting my period. This is, of course, because I no longer experience the surge in hormones produced by the ovaries that would bring about this effect. However, I am not concerned by this; I am simply relieved that I continue to have a desire for sex.

With regard to having undergone a mastectomy, I am delighted by how good my reconstructed breasts look; I continue to feel very womanly, attractive and sexy. However, I miss the softness and the warmth of my natural breasts and I miss the erotic sensation in my nipples, by far the most. This has undoubtedly been my biggest sense of loss. Both of my nipples are numb, as is the skin up to an inch or so surrounding them, with the skin beneath the nipple down to the infra-mammary fold being the numbest area of my breasts. While my breasts are mostly numb, I do feel pressure whenever they are touched and, often, this actually leads to pain. It's not a pleasant sensation at all, but what I will say is that all is not lost. I have normal sensation running between my breasts, along the cleavage line which feels pleasurable and slightly more feeling within one breast, but it is, unfortunately, not the pleasure that the erotic sensation has to offer.

Just over a year after my mastectomy, I went on holiday with my family. Before going away I had decided that I would, just for a short while, remove my bikini top to determine how truly emotionally strong I was. While I was confident that I was fine, I knew that if there was any part of me that wasn't, then going topless would bring this to the fore. Taking my bikini top off on the beach, I felt confident, self-assured (even with my baby stretch marks) and, all in all, amazing! I knew then, without any doubt, that I really was doing okay.

For the first couple of years after my mastectomy, I was so happy to be free of the worry of breast cancer, and so delighted by how well my reconstruction and recovery had gone, that, initially, I didn't feel a particularly strong sense of loss after my mastectomy; the positive emotions seemed to carry me through. However, the more time that passed, the more I began to miss my natural breasts and I started to grieve their loss. There have been times, for example, where I am going about my daily life, feeling perfectly fine, and perhaps I see a young woman with beautiful breasts on TV. Up will come the most intense grief which has, on one occasion, instantly reduced me to tears. While moments like these are distressing, they are, thankfully, rare. I feel that this sense of grief will probably continue throughout life, similar to how the grief of losing a loved one never really goes. But, at moments like this, I try to console myself by remembering that even though I have lost my natural breasts, gone with them also is the very high risk of breast cancer. In all reality, I am very lucky and thinking this way usually helps to ease these difficult emotions.

With regard to my health post-surgery, so far as bone density or my general wellbeing is concerned, all is presently well. To date, I have had a baseline bone density scan and a further one four years post-BSO, both of which, reassuringly, revealed a normal bone density. I continue to have good energy levels and I am able to fulfil the demands of everyday life, as effectively as prior to my surgeries.

During the first couple of years after removal of my ovaries, I experienced a total of three urinary tract infections, all prior to starting the vaginal oestrogen cream. However, with regular use of this cream and with my stress levels having returned to normal, I have not had any further problems of this nature. Interestingly, during a vaginal examination, performed by a gynaecologist nearly three years after having my ovaries removed, the doctor reassured me that there was no sign of vaginal atrophy and he confirmed that the health of my vagina was exactly the same as that of any other woman my age with their ovaries still intact.

As far as the possibility of experiencing long-term pain after mastectomy is concerned, I sometimes experience discomfort on the side of my left breast. However, it's manageable and never requires any pain relief. I have found that overdoing certain tasks, such as cleaning or decorating, aggravates this further but, again, this never requires pain relief and it resolves within a day or so.

Overall, I can hardly believe that I am doing as well as I am, given what my body has endured.

Section V

Although very tough in many ways, this journey has also been a positive experience. It has reminded me of what truly matters in life, along with the importance of my own happiness. One of the nicest positives from this journey is that I have become a more confident and assertive person, with a stronger desire to really live my life to the full and to create many more happy memories with my family and friends. Furthermore, this journey has also brought my husband and me even closer together, when I didn't think that was possible given how close we already were.

22.
A final thought

If you are a BRCA mutation carrier and are currently trying to decide on which strategy is right for you to lower your risk of cancer, I hope that the information within this book empowers you to make the decision that is right for you. Whether you ultimately decide to undergo risk-reducing surgery or not, I hope that sharing my journey with you has shown that you can get through this period of your life and that life does go on afterwards. Maybe you will come across people who do not understand your decision but, in all likelihood, they are ill-informed and, ultimately, are not the ones going through this journey. This is *your* body and *your* life; do what is right for *you*.

While this journey took me to my emotional limits and sometimes beyond, I got through it by taking one day at a time, one appointment at a time and by allowing myself to go through whatever emotions arose. I leant on those around me when I needed the support but, above all, I kept sight of the knowledge that one day this journey would come to an end and life would return to normal. Furthermore, what really kept me strong throughout was reminding myself that, as difficult as this journey was, being diagnosed with cancer would be far worse. I didn't have to have surgery followed by months of chemotherapy, all the while wondering whether the cancer would return and, ultimately, whether I would live or die. I am one of the fortunate ones and focusing on this helped me to keep perspective; it also gave me the strength and the positivity to cope.

Personally, I hold no regrets with the decisions that I have made. It has all been worth it to be where I am now – free of the worry of breast and ovarian cancer – and to have done everything in my power to ensure that I am around for my family. Because of this, and how very different my future might have otherwise been, I consider myself to be one of the luckiest women in the world.

And finally ... having decided that it would be nice to use a silhouette of a woman's body on the front cover of this book, I began to look for suitable images. However, I quickly came to the realisation that using an image of a young model's body that has not been through these surgeries would be misleading. For this reason, and because this book details my personal journey of undergoing risk-reducing surgery, I decided that there would be no better way to illustrate that it is possible to continue to feel womanly, self-assured and confident, than to use a silhouette of my own post-surgery body.

Glossary

Abdominal hysterectomy – surgical removal of the womb through an incision in the lower abdomen.

Acellular dermal matrix (ADM) – a biological, acellular collagen matrix made of foetal bovine dermis, especially developed for reconstructive surgery.

Advanced-stage cancer – a cancer which is large and has spread to other area(s) of the body. (See also Early-stage cancer.)

Alzheimer's disease – an irreversible, progressive brain disorder that slowly destroys memory and thinking skills and, eventually, the ability to carry out the simplest tasks. Alzheimer's disease is the most common cause of Dementia. (See also Dementia.)

Amino acids – organic compounds that combine to form proteins.

Anaplastic large cell lymphoma (ALCL) – a rare type of lymphoma which has been found in the breast tissue in women who have breast implants. The two main forms of lymphoma are Hodgkin lymphoma and non-Hodgkin lymphoma. ALCL is a very rare type of non-Hodgkin lymphoma.

Angiogenesis – the development of new blood vessels.

Areola – a small circular area, in particular the ring of pigmented skin surrounding a nipple.

Areola-sparing mastectomy – a mastectomy which removes the breast tissue and the nipple, but not the areola.

Atypia – a term used to describe cells which look structurally different from normal cells – that is, atypical-looking cells.

Atypical ductal hyperplasia – a benign (not cancer) condition in which the cells lining the breast ducts have increased in number and have developed an unusual pattern or shape. Having atypical ductal hyperplasia has been shown to slightly increase the risk of developing breast cancer in the future.

Augmentation (breast) – a surgical procedure which aims to increase the size, shape or fullness of the breast.

Autosomal dominant inheritance – a pattern of inheritance characteristic of some genetic diseases. 'Autosomal' means that the gene in question is located on one of the numbered, or non-sex, chromosomes. 'Dominant' means that a single copy of the disease-associated mutation is enough to cause the disease.

Basal breast cancer – Basal-like breast cancer tumours are among the most aggressive – they grow fast and spread quickly, making them more likely than other types of cancer to be fatal. These tumours are more likely to be resistant to standard breast cancer treatments, such as tamoxifen or herceptin, making them especially difficult to treat. This type of breast cancer is strongly associated with BRCA1 gene mutations.

Baseline – a starting point used for comparisons, e.g. a baseline bone density scan prior to oophorectomy, which can be used to compare with bone density scans taken after oophorectomy to determine if there has been any loss in bone density. (See also Osteopenia and Osteoporosis).

Benign (of a disease, tumour, etc) – not malignant.

Bilateral – means on 'both sides', e.g. as in a 'bilateral oophorectomy' to remove both ovaries.

Bilateral cancer – a cancer that occurs in both paired organs – for example, both breasts, kidneys, ovaries, whether at the same time or later.

BOCS (The Breast and Ovarian Cancer Susceptibility Study) – aims to identify the genetic factors involved in causing breast and ovarian cancer. For further information, please visit www.icr.ac.uk/our-research/research-divisions/division-of-genetics-and-epidemiology/genetic-

susceptibility/research-projects/the-breast-and-ovarian-cancer-suscep-
tibility-(bocs)-study

Bone densitometry scan – a special type of X-ray test used to measure
the calcium content of the bone. The examination is also called a 'dual
energy X-ray absorptiometry' (DEXA) scan or a 'quantitative digital
radiography' (QDR) scan. The DEXA scan is the established standard
for measuring bone mineral density (BMD).

Bone mineral density (BMD) – a medical term normally referring to the
amount of mineral matter per square centimetre of bones. Bone density
is used in clinical medicine as an indirect indicator of osteoporosis and
fracture risk.

BRCA genes – tumour-suppressor genes which function to prevent the
formation of cancer.

BRCA1 (BReast CAncer gene 1) – a tumour suppressor gene which
produces tumour suppressor proteins which function to prevent the
formation of cancer.

BRCA2 (BReast CAncer gene 2) – a tumour suppressor gene which
produces tumour suppressor proteins which function to prevent the
formation of cancer.

Breast cancer cluster region (BCCR) – the region of a BRCA gene which
is associated with a higher risk of breast cancer and a lower risk of ovarian cancer compared with BRCA mutations which sit outside this region.

Breast Cancer Linkage Consortium – a worldwide cooperative network
of scientists who share a major interest in inherited breast and ovarian
cancer. The BCLC has provided accurate estimates of the cancer risks associated with the BRCA1 and BRCA2 genes, and on the type of families
associated with them. These data are widely used in clinical settings in
which women with a strong positive family history, or those diagnosed
as carrying a defect in these genes, should decide, together with their
health providers, for or against risk-reducing measures.

Breast self-examination – a self-examination which a woman (or a
man) can perform to look for changes in the breast tissue (see page 119).

BSO – see Salpingo-oophorectomy (page 273).

'c.' – **refers to a coding DNA** sequence, such as c.5130_5133delTGTA. (See also Coding DNA.)

Cancer – a condition in which cells in a specific part of the body begin to reproduce uncontrollably.

Cancer antigen 19-9 (CA 19-9) – a protein found on the surface of many pancreatic cancer cells which is used as a tumour marker to help diagnose pancreatic cancer and to monitor pancreatic cancer treatment or recurrence.

Cancer antigen 125 (CA-125) – a protein found on the surface of many ovarian cancer cells which is used as a tumour marker to help diagnose ovarian cancer and to determine if ovarian cancer treatment is working.

Capsular contracture – a breast implant is a foreign body and, like all implanted foreign bodies, the immune system will respond to it by encasing it in a very thin fibrous layer. Often, this capsule will be of no consequence but in some patients, and for reasons unknown, this fibrous layer can become very thick and may contract, squeezing the implant. When this happens, the breast tends to become hard, and more round in appearance, causing discomfort or pain.

Carcinogen – any substance, radionuclide or radiation that is an agent directly involved in causing cancer. This may be due to the ability to damage the genome or to the disruption of cellular metabolic processes.

Carcinoma – a type of cancer that develops from epithelial cells. Specifically, a carcinoma is a cancer that begins in a tissue that lines the inner or outer surfaces of the body.

Carcinomatosis – a condition in which multiple carcinomas develop simultaneously, usually after dissemination from a primary source.

Cell – the basic unit of life. It is the smallest structural and functional unit of an organism, which is typically microscopic and consists of cytoplasm and a nucleus enclosed in a membrane.

Cell division – the process by which a parent cell divides into two or more genetically identical daughter cells.

Cervical dysplasia – a precancerous condition in which abnormal cell growth occurs on the surface lining of the cervix.

CHEK2 – the biggest discovery since BRCA2 has probably been CHEK2 (Checkpoint Kinase 2), first discovered in 2004. Inherited mutations in CHEK2 are associated with a one in two risk of breast cancer up to the age of 80 and may also increase the risk of male breast cancer, prostate cancer, colon cancer and lung cancer. This gene interacts with BRCA1, BRCA2 and TP53 to repair DNA.

Chemoprevention – the use of drugs to prevent or delay the development of cancer.

Chromosomes – thread-like structures located inside the nucleus of animal and plant cells. They are made up of long strands of DNA and they contain an enormous number of genes.

Chronic pain – pain lasting 12 or more weeks. Acute pain is a normal sensation that alerts us to possible injury, but chronic pain persists, often for months or even longer.

Clinical trial – a type of clinical research that compares one treatment with another. It may involve patients or healthy people, or both.

Coding DNA – the portion of a gene's DNA, composed of exons, that codes for the production of a protein – for example, the portion in the BRCA gene which codes for the production of a tumour suppressor protein.

Codon – a sequence of three DNA nucleotides, for example, that corresponds with a specific amino acid or stop signal during protein synthesis.

CRISPR-Cas9 – a genome editing tool that enables geneticists and medical researchers to edit parts of the genome by cutting out, replacing or adding parts to the DNA sequence.

CT scan (computerised tomography scan, also known as a CAT scan) – an imaging method that uses x-rays to create pictures of cross-sections of the body.

Cumulative risk – a measure of the total risk that a certain event will happen during a given period of time.

DCIS (ductal carcinoma in situ) – considered to be the earliest form of breast cancer in which abnormal cells are found in the lining of the breast ducts.

Debulking – as in 'debulking of a tumour', is surgery to remove as much of the tumour as possible.

Delayed-oophorectomy – later removal of ovaries after fallopian tubes have been removed.

Dementia – a set of symptoms that may include memory loss and difficulties with thinking, problem-solving or language. A person with dementia may also experience changes in their mood or behaviour. Dementia is caused when the brain is damaged by diseases, such as Alzheimer's disease or a series of strokes.

Diabetes – a long-term condition in which blood sugar levels are higher than normal.

DIEP flap – a type of breast reconstruction in which blood vessels called 'deep inferior epigastric perforators' (DIEP), as well as the skin and fat connected to them, are removed from the lower abdomen and transferred to the chest to reconstruct a breast after mastectomy, without sacrificing any of the abdominal muscles.

DNA (deoxyribonucleic acid) – the hereditary material in humans and almost all other organisms. Nearly every cell in a person's body has the same DNA.

DTI (direct to implants) breast reconstruction – a post-mastectomy breast reconstruction which allows surgeons to place a breast implant immediately, avoiding the use of a tissue expander. This 'one-step' approach allows patients to awake from their mastectomy with a well-defined breast shape.

Ducts (breast) – small channels responsible for delivering breast milk to the surface of the skin and out through tiny pores in the nipple. These ducts form a tree-branch-like network that converges at the nipple.

Early-stage cancer – a cancer which is small and may not have spread to other area(s) of the body. (See also Advanced-stage cancer.)

EMBRACE (Epidemiological Study of Familial Breast Cancer) study – a major study ongoing in the UK to examine lifestyle and additional genetic factors which may increase or decrease cancer risk in people who are known to carry a BRCA1 or BRCA2 gene mutation. For further information, please visit http://ccge.medschl.cam.ac.uk/embrace/

Endometrial (uterine) cancer – a cancer which begins in the cells that make up the lining of the womb (called the endometrium).

Endometrial hyperplasia – a thickening of the lining of the womb, caused by overgrowth of the cells that line it which may, in turn, increase the risk for endometrial (uterine) cancer.

Endoscopic ultrasound (EUS) – insertion of a tiny scope with an ultrasound probe down the oesophagus (food pipe) to the stomach, allowing examination of oesophageal and stomach linings as well as the walls of the upper and lower gastrointestinal tract. EUS can also be used to study the pancreas.

Epithelial ovarian cancer – the most common form of ovarian cancer, both in the general population and in female BRCA mutation carriers. (See also Serous epithelial ovarian cancer.)

Exon – the portion of the gene's DNA that contains the genetic code for the production of a protein.

Extended latissimus dorsi – skin and latissimus dorsi muscle are taken from the back and used to reconstruct the breast without the use of a breast implant.

Fallopian tubes – a pair of thin tubes which transport a woman's eggs from her ovaries to her uterus (womb) each month where they are either fertilised by sperm or discarded during menstruation.

False negative – a test result improperly indicates no presence of a condition (the result is negative) when in reality it is present.

False positive – a test result improperly indicates the presence of a condition when in reality it isn't present.

Fibroids – benign tumours of the uterus.

Gene – any section along the DNA that carries instructions which allow a cell to produce proteins.

Genetic counselling – a medical specialty in which a counsellor calculates the risk of recurrence of inherited disorders in families, using pedigree charts and applying the laws of inheritance.

Genetic engineering – the deliberate modification of the characteristics of an organism by manipulating its genetic material.

Gene therapy – involves inserting normal genes into cells in place of missing or defective ones in order to correct genetic disorders.

Genome – an organism's complete set of DNA, including all of its genes. Each genome contains all of the information needed to build and maintain that organism. In humans, a copy of the entire genome – more than 3 billion DNA base pairs – is contained in all cells that have a nucleus.

Grade (of a cancer) – the appearance of the cancerous cells under a microscope compared with normal cells and how fast the cancer is growing. (See also high-grade cancer and low-grade cancer).

Gynaecologist – a surgeon who specialises in diseases of the female reproductive systems (vagina, uterus and ovaries, etc).

Gynaecological oncologist – a gynaecologist who specialises in the diagnosis and treatment of women with cancer of the reproductive organs.

HBOC (hereditary breast and ovarian cancer syndromes) – produce higher than normal levels of breast cancer and ovarian cancer in genetically related families (either one individual had both, or several individuals in the family had one or the other cancer).

Heterozygous – having two different forms of a gene. The Greek root 'hetero-' means different', and a zygote is a cell created when two gametes – a sperm and an egg, in humans – come together.

High-grade cancer – a high-grade tumour contains cells which are very abnormal looking, are faster growing and are more likely to have spread. (See also Low-grade cancer.)

Homozygous – having two of the same forms of a gene. The Greek root 'homo-' means 'same', and a zygote is a cell created when two gametes – a sperm and an egg, in humans – come together.

Hot flushes (known also as hot flashes, in the US, for example) – sudden waves of mild or intense body heat, usually in the face, neck and chest, which happen as a reaction to oestrogen deficiency in the blood vessels of the skin, as a symptom of the menopause.

Housekeeping genes – genes that are expressed in all cells of the body and code for proteins that are essential for basic cell growth and metabolism.

HRT (hormone replacement therapy) – a treatment used to relieve the symptoms of the menopause by replacing female hormones that are at a lower level approaching the menopause.

Hypo-active sexual desire disorder – considered to be a sexual dysfunction, characterised as a lack or absence of sexual fantasies and desire for sexual activity.

Hysterectomy – removal of the uterus (womb).

IgG4 – Immunoglobulin G is the main type of antibody found in the blood and it protects against infection within the body. By binding many kinds of pathogens, such as viruses, bacteria and fungi, IgG protects the body from infection and IgG4 is one of four immunoglobulin Gs.

IMF (infra-mammary fold) – the fold at the base of the breast where the breast and the chest meet, through which risk-reducing mastectomies can be performed.

IMPACT study (Identification of Men with a genetic predisposition to ProstAte Cancer: Targeted screening in men at a higher genetic risk and controls) – an international study which aims to discover whether screening to detect prostate cancer can be targeted at men who carry the BRCA1, BRCA2 and Lynch syndrome alterations, leading to earlier diagnosis and improved survival. For further information, please visit www.impact-study.co.uk.

Implant-breast reconstruction – reconstruction using implants.

Inflammatory breast cancer (IBC) – a rare and aggressive form of breast cancer. The breast appears swollen, red, warm and tender rather than forming a lump; the symptoms are similar to those of an infection in the breast.

Invasive – cancer, for example, that is spreading very quickly and undesirably or harmfully.

Lactation – the secretion of milk by the mammary glands.

Laparoscopic surgery (also called 'minimally invasive surgery' (MIS), or 'keyhole surgery') – a type of surgical procedure that allows a surgeon to access the inside of the abdomen (tummy) and pelvis without having to make large incisions in the skin.

Laparotomy – a surgical incision into the abdominal cavity, for diagnosis or in preparation for major surgery.

Latissimus dorsi flap reconstruction – skin and latissimus dorsi muscle are taken from the back and used to reconstruct the breast. In most cases, a breast implant has to be placed under the flap to achieve the desired shape, size and projection.

Libido (colloquially known as 'sex drive') – a person's overall sexual drive or desire for sexual activity.

Low-grade cancer – a low-grade tumour contains cells which look very similar to normal looking cells, but are slower growing and are less likely to have spread than a high-grade one. (See also High-grade cancer.)

Low-stage cancer – a low-stage tumour contains cells which are small and haven't spread anywhere else. (See also Advanced-stage cancer.)

Lymphoedema – a chronic condition that causes swelling when the lymphatic system is not able to drain fluid properly. Many people with breast cancer have at least two or three lymph nodes removed from under the arm (sentinel lymph node biopsy), and sometimes many more nodes (axillary lymph node dissection). If the cancer has spread, it has most likely moved into those underarm lymph nodes first because they drain lymph from the breast tissue.

Lynch syndrome (also called Hereditary nonpolyposis colon cancer (HNPCC)) – a hereditary disorder caused by a mutation in a mismatch repair gene in which affected individuals have a higher than normal chance of developing colorectal cancer, endometrial cancer, and various other types of aggressive cancers, often at a young age.

Magnetic resonance cholangiopancreatography (MRCP) – a special type of magnetic resonance imaging (MRI) examination that produces detailed images of the hepatobiliary and pancreatic systems, including the liver, gallbladder, bile ducts, pancreas and pancreatic duct.

Malignant – if the cells of a tumour are cancerous, the tumour is described as malignant.

Mammogram – a breast X-ray. It can help detect breast cancer before there are any obvious signs or symptoms.

Mammography – a specific type of breast imaging that uses low-dose

X-rays to detect cancer early – before women experience symptoms – when it is most treatable.

Mastectomy – removal of the breast tissue.

Menopause – the end of menstruation when a woman's periods stop permanently and she can no longer become pregnant.

Mesothelial atypia – abnormal-looking cells of the peritoneum.

Meta-analysis – uses a statistical approach to combine the results from multiple studies in an effort to increase power (over individual studies), improve estimates of the size of the effect and/or to resolve uncertainty when reports disagree.

Metastases – tumours resulting from metastasis, or metastatic disease, which is the spread of a cancer or other disease from one organ or part of the body to another.

Micro-metastases – forms of metastases in which the newly formed tumours are too small to be detected.

Mini-pill – contraceptive pill containing progesterone alone.

Mitosis – cell division which produces a genetically identical daughter cell.

Morbidity – the state of being ill or diseased.

Mortality – death.

MRI (magnetic resonance imaging) – a type of scan that uses strong magnetic fields and radio waves to produce detailed images of the inside of the body. It can be used to detect breast cancer before there are any obvious signs or symptoms.

Multi-gene panel testing – genetic testing which simultaneously examines a number of different genes to look for potentially cancer-causing mutations, which can provide information to help people take action to prevent or stop cancer.

Mutation – alteration or change in DNA which may, or may not be, harmful.

National Breast Screening Programme – an NHS population breast screening programme available to all women aged 50-70.

Necrosis – the death of body tissue which occurs when too little blood flows to the tissue. For example, when the breast tissue is removed during mastectomy, some of the nerves and blood vessels are unavoidably removed and if inadequate blood flow remains to the skin, it can lead to the tissue dying as a result of too little oxygen reaching the tissues.

Nerve-sparing mastectomy – is a procedure which maintains the nerves that provide sensation to the skin over the breasts. Breasts that have undergone any of these surgeries have much less tactile sensation than natural breasts. Nerve-sparing techniques are an effort to retain some feeling in the breasts, with limited and often only partial success.

NICE (the National Institute for Health and Care Excellence) – provides national guidance and advice to improve health and social care.

NICE Guidelines – quality standards to improve the quality of the UK's National Health Service (NHS).

Night sweats – hot flushes which occur during the night as a reaction to oestrogen deficiency in the blood vessels of the skin.

Nipple-sparing mastectomy (also called a 'subcutaneous nipple-sparing mastectomy') – a skin-sparing mastectomy which removes the breast tissue, but leaves the nipple and areola intact for a more natural appearance. The scars may be hidden in the inframammary fold under the breast.

Nulliparity/a nulliparous woman – a woman who has never given birth.

Oestrogen – the primary female sex hormone, which is responsible for development and regulation of the female reproductive system and secondary sex characteristics, such as breast development.

Oophorectomy – surgical removal of the ovaries.

Oral contraceptives – medications that prevent pregnancy. They are one method of birth control.

Osteopenia – a condition in which bone mineral density is lower than normal, considered by many doctors to be a precursor to osteoporosis.

Osteoporosis – a medical condition in which the bones become brittle and fragile from loss of tissue, typically as a result of hormonal changes, or deficiency of calcium or vitamin D.

Ovarian cancer cluster region (OCCR) – the region of the BRCA gene which is associated with a higher risk of ovarian cancer and a lower risk of breast cancer compared with BRCA mutations which sit outside this region.

Ovaries – a pair of small organs in the female reproductive system which contain and release an egg once a month. This process is known as ovulation.

Over-diagnosis – the diagnosis and treatment of breast cancer that would never have made a woman ill in her lifetime – she would never have known about it if she had not been screened.

Ovum (egg) freezing – a procedure, typically used for women who are about to undergo cancer treatment, in which a woman's eggs can be retrieved and then frozen with the goal of being used in the future when the patient is ready to start a family.

Pack years – a measure of how much an individual has smoked in the past, calculated by multiplying the number of packs of cigarettes smoked per day by the number of years the person has smoked. For example, one pack-year is equal to smoking 20 cigarettes (one pack) per day for one year.

PALB2 – a partner and localiser of the BRCA2 gene which encodes a protein that may function in tumour suppression.

Pancreas – an organ which produces important hormones, such as insulin, to help regulate blood sugar levels. It also plays a part in digestion, secreting pancreatic juice which assists with the digestion and absorption of nutrients in the small intestine.

Parity – the number of times a woman has given birth to a foetus with a gestational age of 24 weeks or more, regardless of whether the child was alive or stillborn.

Parous/a parous woman – a woman who has given birth.

Pathogenic – capable of causing disease e.g. a pathogenic BRCA gene mutation is one which is capable of causing cancer.

PBM (prophylactic bilateral mastectomy) – the removal of both breasts to reduce the risk of breast cancer.

Pectoralis major (colloquially, 'pecs') – a thick, fan-shaped muscle, situated on the chest.

Peri-menopause – the period of a woman's life shortly before the occurrence of the menopause.

Peritoneal washing – a procedure in which a salt-water solution is used to wash the peritoneal cavity and then is removed to check for cancer cells within the peritoneum. Peritoneal washings are commonly done during surgery for cancer of the ovary and uterus, to see if cancer has spread to the peritoneal cavity.

Peritoneum – a membrane which surrounds the abdominal organs, such as the bowel and the liver. The peritoneum protects the organs and acts as a barrier to infection.

Post-mastectomy pain syndrome (PMPS) – chronic nerve pain after mastectomy (or lumpectomy). The classic signs of PMPS are chest wall pain and tingling down the arm. Pain may also be felt in the shoulder, scar, arm or armpit. Other common complaints include numbness, shooting or pricking pain, or unbearable itching. PMPS is thought to be linked to damage done to the nerves in the armpit and chest during surgery, but the causes are not known.

Predictive genetic tests – tests used to detect faulty gene patterns associated with conditions that appear after birth, often later in life. These tests can be helpful to people who have a family member with a genetic condition, but who have no symptoms, signs or abnormal non-genetic tests consistent with the condition at the time of testing. Predictive testing can identify faulty gene patterns that increase a person's chances of developing conditions with a genetic basis.

Pre-implantation genetic diagnosis (PGD) – a technique used in reproductive medicine to identify genetic defects in embryos created through in vitro fertilisation (IVF). It enables couples at risk of passing on an inherited disorder to decrease the risk of having an affected child significantly.

Previvors™ – survivors of a predisposition (or increased risk) for a disease such as cancer.

Primary peritoneal cancer (PPC) – a cancer which develops from cells that form the membrane, known as the peritoneum, which surrounds the abdominal organs.

Progesterone – belongs to a group of steroid hormones called progestogens. It is mainly secreted by the ovary during the second half of the menstrual cycle. It plays important roles in the menstrual cycle and in maintaining the early stages of pregnancy.

Proliferation – rapid increase in the number of, for example, cells.

Prophylactic – a medication or a treatment designed and used to prevent a disease from occurring e.g. prophylactic surgery to prevent cancer.

Prophylactic (preventative) surgery – please see Risk-reducing surgery.

Prostate – a small gland about the size of a walnut which is found below the bladder. It surrounds the first part of the tube (urethra), which carries urine from the bladder to the penis. The same tube also carries semen. The prostate gland is divided into two lobes, to the left and the right of a central groove, and produces a thick clear fluid that is an important part of the semen.

Prostatectomy – a surgical operation to remove all or part of the prostate, common in prostate cancer.

Raloxifene – raloxifene hydrochloride is a medicine used in preventing and treating osteoporosis in women after the menopause.

Regional anaesthetic – an anaesthesiologist makes an injection near a cluster of nerves to numb the area of the body that requires surgery, such as a regional anaesthetic given to the chest to help manage pain after mastectomy.

Risk factor (for cancer) – a risk factor is anything that can increase the chance of developing cancer.

Risk-reducing surgery – surgery to remove healthy tissue which is at high risk of developing cancer, such as the breasts and ovaries in BRCA mutation carriers.

RRSO (risk-reducing salpingo-oophorectomy) – typically performed bilaterally, the surgical removal of ovaries and fallopian tubes to lower the risk of ovarian and fallopian tube cancer.

Salpingectomy – the surgical removal of one or both fallopian tubes. It is often performed in cases of tubal pregnancies (pregnancies which have developed within the fallopian tubes), but can form part of a salpingo-oophorectomy operation to prevent ovarian cancer.

Salpingo-oophorectomy – the surgical removal of a fallopian tube and an ovary. If both sets of fallopian tubes and ovaries are removed, the procedure is called a bilateral salpingo-oophorectomy (BSO).

Screening – the testing of a person or group of people for the presence of a disease or other condition.

Serous epithelial ovarian cancer – a type of epithelial cancer typically seen in BRCA mutation carriers. (See also Epithelial ovarian cancer.)

Sexuality – capacity for sexual feelings.

Simple mastectomy – removes all of the breast tissue and most of the skin covering the breasts, leaving the least amount of breast tissue in the body; therefore, achieving the greatest risk reduction. It may be recommended for women not having breast reconstruction. In addition to risk-reducing use, it is also used by women who have been diagnosed with earlier stages of cancer.

Skin-sparing mastectomy – removes all of the breast tissue, including the nipple and areola, but leaves the 'excess' skin in place for reconstruction. It has less visible scar tissue than a simple mastectomy.

Stage (of a cancer) – describes the size of a tumour and how far it has spread from where it originated. (See also Advanced-stage cancer and Early-stage cancer.)

Tamoxifen (tamoxifen citrate) – a drug which blocks the actions of oestrogen and is used to treat and prevent some types of breast cancer.

Testosterone – the principal male sex hormone responsible for the development of the male reproductive system and secondary sexual characteristics, such as increased muscle, bone mass, and the growth of body hair. Testosterone is also produced in women, albeit to a lesser extent.

Tissue expander implant breast reconstruction – a staged breast reconstruction begins with a tissue expander at the time of mastectomy, followed by placement of the final implant at a second stage. The tissue expander itself is essentially a pouch that can be expanded by injection of saline through a self-sealing port. Once the desired volume is achieved, the second stage of reconstruction, which involves replacing the tissue expander with a breast implant, can be planned.

TNBC (triple-negative breast cancer) – breast cancer that has not grown in response to the hormones oestrogen or progesterone or the protein HER2. It accounts for up to 15% of women with breast cancer and is more common in younger, pre-menstrual women.

Tomosynthesis – a special kind of mammogram that produces a three-dimensional image of the breast by using several low-dose X-rays obtained at different angles.

Total abdominal hysterectomy with bilateral salpingo-oophorectomy (TAH BSO) – removal of the womb, cervix, fallopian tubes (salpingectomy) and ovaries (oophorectomy).

Total hysterectomy – removal of both the uterus (womb) and cervix; it is the most commonly performed type of hysterectomy.

TP53 – a tumour-suppressor gene which gives instructions for making a protein called p53 that helps stop the growth of abnormal cells. If this gene carries a harmful mutation, it can lose its tumour-suppressor function.

Tram flap reconstruction – the transverse *rectus abdominis* muscle, which lies in the lower abdomen, is used to reconstruct the breast.

Tubal ligation (or 'tubectomy', also known as 'having one's tubes tied') – a surgical procedure for sterilisation in which a woman's fallopian tubes are clamped and blocked, or severed and sealed; whichever method is used, it prevents an egg from reaching the uterus for implantation.

UKCTOCS (UK Collaborative Trial of Ovarian Cancer Screening) – the world's largest ovarian cancer-screening trial looking at whether screening tests would be useful for diagnosing ovarian cancer in the general population and if screening can save lives. For further information, please see www.ucl.ac.uk/womens-health/research/womens-cancer/gynaecological-cancer-research-centre/ukctocs

UK FOCSS (the UK Familial Ovarian Cancer Screening Study) – looked at ovarian cancer screening in high-risk women. Its aim was to find out which screening tests would be best for women at high risk of ovarian cancer and to determine how often women should be screened. For further information, please visit www.ucl.ac.uk/womens-health/research/womens-cancer/gynaecological-cancer-research-centre/ukfocss

Ultrasound scan (also called a 'sonogram', 'diagnostic sonography' and 'ultrasonography') – a technique that uses high-frequency sound waves to create an image of some part of the inside of the body, such as a foetal ultrasound scan used to monitor an unborn baby.

Unilateral – means 'one-sided' – such as a 'unilateral mastectomy', removal of only one breast.

Uterine serous carcinoma (USC) (also known as 'uterine papillary serous carcinoma' (UPSC) – an aggressive type of uterine cancer which, under the microscope, resembles the fallopian tube cancers and ovarian cancers seen in female BRCA mutation carriers.

Uterus (also known as the 'womb') – a hollow, muscular organ of the female reproductive system which is responsible for the development of the embryo and foetus during pregnancy and for pushing the baby out when it reaches term.

Vaginal atrophy – the thinning of the walls of the vagina caused by decreased oestrogen levels, most commonly associated with menopause. Symptoms may include redness, itching and dryness. Over time, there may be narrowing and shrinkage of the vaginal opening and the vagina itself. The atrophy can also spread to the urinary tract, leading to difficulty urinating, bloody urine and other problems.

Vaginal dryness (also known as 'atrophic vaginitis') – deficiency or absence of vaginal lubrication during sexual activity, often caused by decreased levels of the hormone oestrogen during the menopause.

Vaginal hysterectomy – a surgical procedure in which the uterus and cervix are removed through the vagina. Because it is less invasive than a traditional hysterectomy, recovery is often much faster.

Vaginal prolapse – a condition in which structures such as the uterus, rectum, bladder, urethra, small bowel or vagina itself may begin to 'prolapse', or fall out of their normal positions; they may even protrude out of the body through the vaginal opening, usually following menopause, childbirth or a hysterectomy.

Vaginal vault prolapse – a prolapse in which the top of the vagina falls towards the vaginal opening. This may cause the walls of the vagina to weaken as well and the top of the vagina may protrude out of the body through the vaginal opening, effectively turning the vagina inside out. This condition is common after hysterectomy, with upwards of 10% of women developing some degree of vaginal vault prolapse after surgery.

Variants of uncertain significance (VUS) (also known as 'variants of unknown significance' or 'unclassified variant') – a mutation in the DNA of a gene whose association with disease risk is unknown.

Wild-type – the normal, non-mutated version of a gene common in nature. For example, BRCA genes which do not carry a mutation are described as 'wild-type BRCA1/2'.

Appendix
European BRCA1/2 mutations

Most common and founder BRCA1/2 mutations in European populations:

Population	BRCA1 mutation	
	HGVS	**BIC**
Ashkenazi Jews	c.68_69delAG	185delAG
	c.5266dupC	5382insC
Austrian	c.181T>G	300T>G
	c.5266dupC	5382insC
	c.1687C>T	1806C>T
	c.3016_3019del4	3135del4
	c.2676_2679del4	2795del4
Slovenian	c.1687C>T	1806C>T
	c.181T>G	300T>G
	c.5266dupC	5382insC
	c.181T>A	300T>A
Italian (Tuscany)	c.3228_3229delAG	3347delAG
	c.3285delA	3404delA
	c.1380dupA	1499insA
	c.5062_5064del3	5181delGTT
Italian (Calabria)	c.4964_4982del19	5083del19
Italian (North-East)	c.5062_5064delGTT	5181_5183delGTT

French	c.3481_3491del11	3600del11
	c.5128G>T	5247G>T
Spanish	c.68_69delAG	185delAG
	c.211A>G (Galicia)	330A>G
	c.5117G>A	5236G>A
	c.5123C>A	5242C>A
	c.470_471delCT	589_590delCT
	c.5153-1G>A	5272-1G>A
Belgian	c.212+3A>G	IVS5+3A>G
	c.2359dupG	2478insG
	c.3661G>T	3780G>T
Dutch	c.2685_2686delAA	2804delAA
	c.2193del5	2312del5
	c.1292dupT	1411insT
	exon 13 deletion (3,8-kb)	
	exon 22 deletion (510-bp)	
German	exon 17 deletion	
	c.5266dupC	5382insC
	c.181T>G	300T>G
	c.4065_4068del4	4184del4
	c.2338C>T	2457C>T
Czech	c.181T>G	300T>G
	c.5266dupC	5382insC
	c.3700_3704del5	3819del5
	exons 1–17 deletion	
	exons 5–14 deletion	
Hungarian	c.5266dupC	5382insC
	c.181T>G	300T>G
	c.68_69delAG	185delAG

Appendix

Greek	c.5266dupC	5382insC
	c.5212G>A	5331G>A
	c.5251C>T	5370C>T
	c.5467G>A	5586G>A
Danish	c.2475delC	2594delC
	c.3319G>T	3438G>T
	c.5266dupC	5382insC
	c.3710delT	3829delT
	exons 3-16 deletion	
Swedish	c.3171_3175dup	3171ins5
	c.2475delC	2594delC
	c.1082_1092del11	1201del11
	c.1687C>T	1806C>T
	c.3626delT (Northern)	3745delT
	c.1016dupA	1135insA
	exon 13 duplication (ins6kbEx13)	
Norwegian	c.1556delA	1675delA
	c.3228delAG	3347delAG
	c.697delGT	816delGT
	c.1016dupA	1135insA
	c.3178G>T	3297G>T
	c.4745delA	4864delA
	c.2351del7	2470del7
	c.3084del11	3203del11
	c.1A>C	120A>C
	c.5075-2A>C	IVS17-2A>C
	exons 1-13 deletion	
	exon 13 duplication (ins6kbEx13)	

Finnish	c.4097-2A>G	4216-2A>G
	c.3485delA	3604delA
	c.3626delT	3745delT
	c.4327C>T	4446C>T
	c.2684del2	2803delAA
	c.5251C>T	5370C>T
	c.4096+3A>G	IVS11+3A>G
British	c.2681_2682delAA (Scotland)	2800delAA
	c.4065_4068del4 (North-West)	4184del4
	exon 13 duplication (ins6kbEx13)	
Irish	c.427G>T	546G>T
Polish	c.5266dupC	5382insC
	c.181T>G	300T>G
	c.4035delA	4154delA
Latvian	c.4035delA	4154delA
	c.5266dupC	5382insC
Lithuanian	c.4035delA	4154delA
	c.5266dupC	5382insC
Belarusian	c.5266dupC	5382insC
	c.181T>G	300T>G
Russian	c.5266dupC	5382insC

Population	BRCA2 mutation	
	HGVS	BIC
Ashkenazi Jews	c.5946delT	6174delT
Austrian	c.8363G>A	8591G>A
	c.8754+1G>A	IVS21-1G>A
	c.3860delA	4088delA
Slovenian	c.7806-2A>G	IVS16-2A>G
Italian	c.8537_8538delAG (Sardinia)	8765delAG

Appendix

Spanish	c.2808_2811del4 (Castilla-Leon)	3036_3039del4
	c.6629_6630delAA	c.6857delAA
	c.9026_9030del5	9254-9258del5
	c.9310_9311delAA	9538delAA
	c.5146_5149del4	374delTATG
Portuguese	c.156_157insAlu	384insAlu
Belgian	c.516+1G>A	IVS6+1G>A
	c.6275_6276delTT	6503_6504delTT
	c.8904delC	9132delC
Dutch	c.5351dupA	5579insA
	c.6275_6276delTT	6503delTT
German	c.1813dupA	2041insA
	c.4478del4	4706del4
	c.9098dupA	9326insA
Czech	c.7913_7917del5	8141del5
	c.8537_8538del2	8765delAG
Hungarian	c.9098dupA	9326insA
	c.5946delT	6174delT
Cypriot	c.8755delG	8984delG
Danish	c.6373delA	6601delA
	c.1310_1013del4	1538del4
	c.6486_6489del4	6714del4
	c.3847_3848delGT	4075delGT
Swedish	c.4258delG	4486delG
Norwegian	c.2808del4	3036del4
	c.3847delGT	4075delGT
Finnish	c.771_775del5	999del5
	c.7480C>T	7708C>T
	c.8327T>G	8555T>G
	c.9118-2A>G	9346-2A>G
	c.9117+1G>A	9345+1G>A

Iceland	c.771_775del5	999del5
British	c.6275_6276delTT (Scotland)	6503delTT
	c.1929delG (North-West)	2157delG

Courtesy of: Janavičius R et al. Founder BRCA1/2 mutations in the Europe: implications for hereditary breast-ovarian cancer prevention and control. *EPMA J* 2010; 1(3): 397-412.

References

Introduction and Section I: Living with BRCA gene mutations

1. The Royal Marsden Hospital, www.royalmarsden.nhs.uk/sites/default/files/files_trust/brca_0.pdf – The Royal Marsden's: A Beginner's Guide to BRCA1 and BRCA2. Accessed Dec 2016.
2. www.discoverymedicine.com/Steven-A-Narod/2009/07/16/brca1-and-brca2-in-2005/. Accessed Oct 2015.
3. Petrucelli N, Daly MB, Feldman GL. Hereditary breast and ovarian cancer due to mutations in BRCA1 and BRCA2. *Genetics in Medicine* 2010; 12: 245–259.
4. www.nhs.uk/Conditions/predictive-genetic-tests-cancer/Pages/Introduction.aspx. Accessed Dec 2015.
5. www.knowbrca.org/Learn/brca1-and-brca2-gene-mutations. Accessed Dec 2015.
6. www.acog.org/Patients/FAQs/BRCA1-and-BRCA2-Mutations. Accessed Sep 2015.
7. www.kantrowitz.com/kantrowitz/brca.html, Breast Cancer Susceptibility Genes (BRCA), A Public Service of Mark Kantrowitz. Accessed Dec 2015.

Section II: Understanding BRCA gene mutations

1. The Human Karyotype, Courtesy of Nottingham Cytogenetics Laboratory.
2. http://ghr.nlm.nih.gov/handbook/basics/gene. What is a Gene? Accessed Dec 2015.

3. www.medscape.com/viewarticle/842748. BRCA Cancer Risk Differs With Type and Location of Mutations, Ricki Lewis, PhD, April 07, 2015. Accessed Aug 2016.

4. Domchek SM, Tang J, Stopfer J, et al. Biallelic deleterious BRCA1 mutations in a woman with early-onset ovarian cancer. *Cancer* 2013; 3(4): 399-405.

5. Wong-Brown M, McPhillips M, Gleeson M et al. When is a mutation not a mutation: the case of the c.594-2A>C splice variant in a woman harbouring another BRCA1 mutation in trans. *Hered Cancer Clin Pract* 2016; 14: 6.

6. www.kantrowitz.com/kantrowitz/brca.html, Breast Cancer Susceptibility Genes (BRCA), A Public Service of Mark Kantrowitz. Accessed Dec 2015.

7. National Cancer Institute, www.cancer.gov/about-cancer/causes-prevention/genetics/brca-fact-sheet. Accessed Mar 2017.

8. Maeshima Y, Oseto K, Katsuragi R et al. Experience with Bilateral Risk-Reducing Mastectomy for an Unaffected BRCA Mutation Carrier. *J Breast Cancer* 2016; 19(2): 218–221.

9. Ramus SJ, Gayther SA. The contribution of BRCA1 and BRCA2 to ovarian cancer. *Mol Oncol* 2009; 3:138–150.

10. Widschwendter M, Rosenthal AN, Philpott S, et al. The sex hormone system in carriers of BRCA1/2 mutations: a case-control study. *Lancet Oncol* 2013; 14(12): 1226-1232.

11. The Royal Marsden Hospital, www.royalmarsden.nhs.uk/sites/default/files/files_trust/brca_0.pdf – The Royal Marsden's: A Beginner's Guide to BRCA1 and BRCA2. Accessed Dec 2016.

12. Primary breast cancer: ESMO Clinical Practice Guidelines for diagnosis, treatment and follow-up; *European Society for Medical Oncology* (2011).

13. Cancer Research UK, www.cancerresearchuk.org/about-cancer/causes-of-cancer/inherited-cancer-genes-and-increased-cancer-risk/inherited-genes-and-cancer-types#inherited_genes4. Accessed Nov 2015.

14. Litton JK, Ready K, Chen H, et al. Earlier age of onset of BRCA mutation-related cancers in subsequent generations. *Cancer* 2012; 118(2): 321–325.

15. Struewing JP, Hartge P, Wacholder S, et al. The risk of cancer associated with specific mutations of BRCA1 and BRCA2 among

Ashkenazi Jews. *N Engl J Med* 1997; 336(20): 1401-1408.

16. Finkelman BS, et al. Breast and ovarian cancer risk and risk reduction in Jewish BRCA1/2 mutation carriers. *J Clin Oncol* 2012; 30(12): 1321-1328.

17. Lubinski J, Phelan CM, Ghadirian P et al. Cancer variation associated with the position of the mutation in the BRCA2 gene. *Fam Cancer* 2004; 3(1): 1-10.

18. Rebbeck TR, Mitra N, Wan F et al. Association of Type and Location of BRCA1 andBRCA2 Mutations With Risk of Breast and Ovarian Cancer. *JAMA* 2015; 313(13): 1347-1361.

19. Thompson D, Easton D. Breast Cancer Linkage Consortium. Variation in cancer risks, by mutation position, in BRCA2 mutation carriers. *Am J Hum Genet* 2001; 68: 410–419.

20. Cochran G, Hardy, J, Harpending, H. Natural history of Ashkenazi intelligence. *Journal of biosocial science* 2006; 38(5): 659–693 http://harpending.humanevo.utah.edu/Documents/ashkiq.webpub.pdf. Accessed May 2016.

21. Wade N. Researchers Say Intelligence and Diseases May Be Linked in Ashkenazic Genes. *The New York Times*, June 3, 2005. Accessed May 2016.

22. www.cancernetwork.com/articles/possible-evolutionary-advantage-seen-breast-cancer-genes. Possible Evolutionary Advantage Seen in Breast Cancer Genes. Accessed Jul 2015.

23. www.huntsmancancer.org/about/annual-reports/past-reports/2012-annual-report/effects-of-brca-mutations-on-female-fertility.php. Accessed Jul 2015.

24. Oktay K, Moy F, Titus S, Stobezki R, Turan V, Dickler M, Goswami S. Age-related decline in DNA repair function explains diminished ovarian reserve, earlier menopause, and possible oocyte vulnerability to chemotherapy in women with BRCA mutations. *J Clin Oncol* 2014; 32: 1093–1094.

25. Phillips KA et al. Anti- Müllerian Hormone Serum Concentrations of Women With Germline BRCA1 or BRCA2 Mutations. *Human Reproduction.* 2016; 31(5): 1126-1132.

Section III: Cancer and its relationship with BRCA gene mutations

1. Cancer Research UK, www.cancerresearchuk.org/health-professional/cancer-statistics/risk/lifetime-risk. Accessed Dec 2015.
2. BBC News, www.bbc.co.uk/news/health-35591176. Cancer cases rise in UK, says charity. 17 February 2016. Accessed Dec 2016.
3. Cancer Research UK, www.cancerresearchuk.org/about-cancer/what-is-cancer/how-cancers-grow. Accessed Dec 2016.
4. Cancer Research UK, www.cancerresearchuk.org/about-cancer/what-is-cancer. Accessed Dec 2016.
5. Cancer Research UK, www.cancerresearchuk.org/about-cancer/what-is-cancer/how-cancer-can-spread. Accessed Dec 2016.
6. Cancer Research UK, www.cancerresearchuk.org/health-professional/cancer-statistics/incidence/common-cancers-compared#heading-Two. Accessed Feb 2017.
7. Torre LA, Bray F, Siegal RL, et al. Global Cancer Statistics, 2012. *CA Cancer J Clin* 2015; 65(2): 87-108.
8. Breast Cancer Care, www.breastcancercare.org.uk/about-us/media/press-pack-breast-cancer-awareness-month/facts-statistics, Facts and Statistics 2016. Accessed Jan 2017.
9. The American Cancer Society, www.cancer.org/cancer/breastcancer/detailedguide/breast-cancer-key-statistics. Accessed Jan 2017.
10. www.breasthealthuk.com/about-breast-cancer/breast-cancer-survival-rates, Breast Cancer survival rates. Accessed Sep 2016.
11. Cancer Research UK, www.cancerresearchuk.org/health-professional/cancer-statistics/statistics-by-cancer-type/breast-cancer/survival#heading-Zero. Accessed Sep 2016.
12. The Royal Marsden Hospital, www.royalmarsden.nhs.uk/sites/default/files/files_trust/brca_0.pdf – The Royal Marsden's: A Beginner's Guide to BRCA1 and BRCA2. Accessed Dec 2016.
13. Maeshima Y, Oseto K, Katsuragi R et al. Experience with Bilateral Risk-Reducing Mastectomy for an Unaffected BRCA Mutation Carrier. *J Breast Cancer* 2016; 19(2): 218–221.
14. Budroni M et al. Role of BRCA2 mutation status on overall survival among breast cancer patients from Sardinia. *BMC Cancer* 2009; 9: 62: 1471-2407.

15. Verhoog LC, Brekelmans CT, Seynaeve C et al. Survival and tumour characteristics of breast-cancer patients with germline mutations of BRCA1. *Lancet* 1998; 351(9099): 316-321.

16. WHO World Cancer Report 2003, Lyon, France: International Agency for Research on Cancer, www.iarc.fr/en/publications/ pdfs-online/wcr/2003/WorldCancerReport.pdf. Accessed Nov 2015.

17. Adapted from Cancer Research UK, www.cancerresearchuk.org/ about-cancer/breast-cancer/risks-causes/risk-factors. Accessed Feb 2017.

18. Cullinane CA, Lubinski J, Neuhausen SL et al. Effect of pregnancy as a risk factor for breast cancer in BRCA1/BRCA2 mutation carriers. *Int J Cancer* 2005; 117: 988-991.

19. Fishman A. The effects of parity, breastfeeding, and infertility treatment on the risk of hereditary breast and ovarian cancer: a review. *Int J Gynecol Cancer* 2010: 20(11 Suppl 2): S31–33.

20. Kotsopoulos J, Lubinski J, Lynch HT et al. Age at first birth and the risk of breast cancer in BRCA1 and BRCA2 mutation carriers. *Breast Cancer Research and Treatment* 2007; 105(2): 221-228.

21. Pan H, He Z, Ling L et al. Reproductive factors and breast cancer risk among BRCA1 or BRCA2 mutation carriers: results from ten studies. *Cancer Epidemiol* 2014; 38(1): 1-8.

22. Collaborative Group on Hormonal Factors in Breast Cancer. Breast cancer and breastfeeding: collaborative reanalysis of individual data from 47 epidemiological studies in 30 countries, including 50302 women with breast cancer and 96973 women without the disease. *Lancet* 2002; 360: 187–195.

23. Kotsopoulos J, Lubinski J, Salmena L et al. Breastfeeding and the risk of breast cancer in BRCA1 and BRCA2 mutation carriers. *Breast Cancer Res* 2012; 14: R42.

24. Iodice S, Barile M, Rotmensz N et al. Oral contraceptive use and breast or ovarian cancer risk in BRCA1/2 carriers: a meta-analysis. *Eur J Cancer* 2010; 46 (12): 2275-2284.

25. Chlebowski RT, Hendrix SL, Langer RD et al. Influence of estrogen plus progestin on breast cancer and mammography in healthy postmenopausal women: the Women's Health Initiative Randomized Trial. *JAMA* 2003; 289(24): 3243-3253.

26. Rebbeck TR, Friebel T, Wagner T et al. Effect of short-term hormone

replacement therapy on breast cancer risk reduction after bilateral prophylactic oophorectomy in BRCA1 and BRCA2 mutation carriers: the PROSE Study Group. *J Clin Oncol* 2005; 23(31): 7804-7810.

27. Cancer Research UK, www.cancerresearchuk.org/about-cancer/ type/breast-cancer/about/types/dcis-ductal-carcinoma-in-situ. Accessed Feb 2017.

28. Breastcancer.org, www.breastcancer.org/symptoms/types/dcis. Accessed Feb 2017.

29. Cancer Research UK, www.cancerresearchuk.org/health-professional/cancer-statistics/statistics-by-cancer-type/breast-cancer. Accessed Feb 2017.

30. BreastCancer.org, www.breastcancer.org/symptoms/types/ilc. Accessed Feb 2017.

31. www.webmd.com/breast-cancer/guide/invasive-breast-cancer. Accessed Mar 2016.

32. Badve S, Dabbs DJ, Schnitt SJ et al. Basal-like and triple-negative breast cancers: a critical review with an emphasis on the implications for pathologists and oncologists. *Mod Pathol* 2011; 24(2): 157-167.

33. ACMG Translating Genes Into Health, http://acmg.omnibooksonline. com/2010/data/papers/018.pdf. Accessed May 2016.

34. www.webmd.com/breast-cancer/breast-cancer-types-er-positive-her2-positive#1. Accessed Aug 2015.

35. Gonzalez-Angulo M, Chen H, Timms K et al. Incidence and outcome of BRCA mutation carriers with triple receptor-negative breast cancer (TNBC). Presented at the 2010 Breast Cancer Symposium, Washington, DC, October 1-3, 2010. Abstract 160.

36. Breast Cancer Care, www.breastcancercare.org.uk/information-support/have-i-got-breast-cancer/breast-cancer-in-men, Breast cancer in men. Accessed Jan 2017.

37. www.cancer.org/cancer/breast-cancer-in-men/about/key-statistics.html. Accessed Jan 2017.

38. Tai YC, Domchek S, Parmigiani G, Chen S. Breast cancer risk among male BRCA1 and BRCA2 mutation carriers. *J Natl Cancer Inst* 2007; 99(23): 1811-1814.

39. Cancer Research UK, www.cancerresearchuk.org/about-cancer/ type/rare-cancers/rare-cancers-name/breast-cancer-in-men. Accessed May 2016.

References

40. Giordano SH, Cohen DS, Buzdar AU, Perkins G, Hortobagyi GN. Breast carcinoma in men: a population-based study. *Cancer* 2004; 101: 51–57.
41. The American Cancer Society, www.cancer.org/cancer/breastcancerinmen/detailedguide/breast-cancer-in-men-what-is-breast-cancer-in-men. Accessed Jul 2015.
42. Jacobs IJ, Menon U, Ryan A. Ovarian cancer screening and mortality in the UK Collaborative Trial of Ovarian Cancer Screening (UKCTOCS): a randomised controlled trial. *Lancet* 2016; 387: 945-956.
43. Ramus SJ, et al. Germline Mutations in the BRIP1, BARD1, PALB2, and NBN Genes in Women With Ovarian Cancer. *J Natl Cancer Inst* 2015; 107(11). doi:10.1093/jnci/djv214
44. www.cancerresearchuk.org/about-us/cancer-news/press-release/2016-01-19-scientists-find-new-gene-fault-behind-ovarian-cancer. Accessed Mar 2017.
45. Cancer Research UK, www.cancerresearchuk.org/about-cancer/causes-of-cancer/inherited-cancer-genes-and-increased-cancer-risk/inherited-genes-and-cancer-types#inherited_genes4. Accessed Nov 2015.
46. Ramus SJ, Gayther SA. The contribution of BRCA1 and BRCA2 to ovarian cancer. *Mol Oncol* 2009; 3: 138–150.
47. Cancer Research UK, www.cancerresearchuk.org/about-cancer/type/ovarian-cancer/about/ovarian-cancer-risks-and-causes. Accessed Sep 2015.
48. McGuire V, Felberg A, Mills M et al. Relation of contraceptive and reproductive history to ovarian cancer risk in carriers and noncarriers of BRCA1 gene mutations. *Am J Epidemiol* 2004;160: 613-618.
49. McLaughlin JR, Risch HA, Lubinski J et al. Reproductive risk factors for ovarian cancer in carriers of BRCA1 or BRCA2 mutations: a case control study. *Lancet Oncol* 2007; 8: 26-34.
50. Antoniou AC, Rookus M, Andrieu N et al. Reproductive and hormonal Factors, and ovarian cancer risk for BRCA1 and BRCA2 mutation carriers: results from the International BRCA1/2 Carrier Cohort Study. *Cancer Epidemiol Biomarkers Prev* 2009; 18: 601-610.
51. Collaborative Group on Epidemiological Studies of Ovarian Cancer, Beral V, Doll R, Hermon C et al. Ovarian cancer and

oral contraceptives: collaborative reanalysis of data from 45 epidemiological studies including 23,257 women with ovarian cancer and 87,303 controls. *Lancet* 2008; 371(9609): 303-314.

52. Cancer Research UK, www.cancerresearchuk.org/sites/default/files/achieving_world-class_cancer_outcomes_-_a_strategy_for_england_2015-2020.pdf. Accessed Feb 2017.

53. Girolimetti G,Perrone AM, Santini D et al. BRCA-Associated Ovarian Cancer: From Molecular Genetics to Risk Management. *Biomed Res Int* 2014; 2014: 787143.

54. Antoniou A, Pharoah PDP, Narod S et al. Average risks of breast and ovarian cancer associated with mutations in BRCA1 or BRCA2 detected in case series unselected for family history: a combined analysis of 22 studies. *Am J Hum Genet* 2003; 72: 1117-1130.

55. Bolton KL, Chenevix-Trench G, Goh C et al. Association between BRCA1 and BRCA2 mutations and survival in women with invasive epithelial ovarian cancer. *Journal of the American Medical Association* 2012; 307(4): 382–390.

56. Brose MS, Rebbeck TR, Calzone KA et al. Cancer Risk Estimates for BRCA1 Mutation Carriers Identified in a Risk Evaluation Program. Oxford Journals. *Medicine & Health JNCI J Natl Cancer Inst* 2002; 94 (18): 1365-1372.

57. Levine DA, Argenta PA, Yee CJ et al. Fallopian tube and primary peritoneal carcinomas associated with BRCA mutations. *J Clin Oncol* 2003; 21(22): 4222-4227.

58. Callahan MJ, Crum CP, Medeiros F et al. Primary fallopian tube malignancies in BRCA-positive women undergoing surgery for ovarian cancer risk reduction. *J Clin Oncol* 2007; 25(25): 3985-3990.

59. Fallopian Tube Cancer: The Basics. www.oncolink.org/types/article.cfm?c=438&id=9502. Accessed Nov 2015.

60. Cass I, Holschneider C, Datta N, Barbuto D, Walts AE, Karlan BY. BRCA-mutation-associated fallopian tube carcinoma: a distinct clinical phenotype? *Obstet Gynecol* 2005; 106(6): 1327-1334.

61. www.cancer.net/cancer-types/ovarian-fallopian-tube-and-peritoneal-cancer/statistics, Ovarian, Fallopian Tube, and Peritoneal Cancer: Statistics. Accessed Sep 2016.

62. Casey MJ, Synder C, Bewtra C, et al. Intra-abdominal carcinomatosis after prophylactic oophorectomy in women of hereditary breast ovarian cancer syndrome kindreds associated with BRCA1 and

BRCA2 mutations. *Gynecol Oncol* 2005; 97(2): 457-467.

63. Eitan R, Soslow R, Lin O, Kauff ND, Liu L, Barakat RR, Chi DS. The significance of cytological mesothelial atypia diagnosed from peritoneal washings performed during risk-reducing salpingo-oophorectomy. *Gynecol Oncol* 2006; 102(2): 315-318.

64. Haldar K, Giamougiannis P, Crawford R. Utility of peritoneal lavage cytology during laparoscopic salpingo-oophorectomy: a retrospective analysis. *BJOG* 2011; 118(1): 28-33.

65. Facing Our Risk of Cancer Empowered (FORCE), www.facingourrisk.org/understanding-brca-and-hboc/information/risk-management/oophorectomy/basics/choice-of-surgeons.php#text. Surgical Removal of Ovaries and Tubes. Accessed Sep 2016.

66. Cancer Research UK, www.cancerresearchuk.org/about-cancer/womb-cancer/risks-causes, Accessed Mar 2017.

67. Lu KH. Management of early-stage endometrial cancer. *Semin Oncol* 2009; 36(2): 137-144.

68. Lavie O, Ben-Arie A, Segev Y et al. BRCA Germline Mutations in Women With Uterine Serous Carcinoma-Still a Debate. *International Journal of Gynecological Cancer* 2010; 20(9): 1531-1534.

69. Goshen R, Chu W et al. Is uterine papillary serous adenocarcinoma a manifestation of the hereditary breast-ovarian cancer syndrome? *Gynecol Oncol* 2000; 79(3): 477-481.

70. Levine DA, Lin O, Barakat RR et al. Risk of endometrial carcinoma associated with BRCA mutation. *Gynecol Oncol* 2001; 80: 395-398.

71. Thompson D, Easton DF. Breast Cancer Linkage Consortium. Cancer incidence in BRCA1 mutation carriers. *J Natl Cancer Inst.* 2002; 94(18): 1358-1365.

72. Segev Y, Iqbal J, Lubinski J et al. Hereditary Breast Cancer Study Group. The incidence of endometrial cancer in women with BRCA1 and BRCA2 mutations. *Gynecol Oncol* 2013; 130(1): 127-131.

73. Shu CA, Pike M, Jotwani AR et al. Risk of developing uterine corpus cancer (Ut Ca) following risk-reducing salpingo-oophorectomy (RRSO) in women with BRCA mutations. Society of Gynecologic Oncology (SGO) Annual Meeting; March 24, 2014.

74. Shu CA, Pike MC, Jotwani AR et al. Uterine Cancer After Risk-Reducing Salpingo-oophorectomy Without Hysterectomy in Women With BRCA Mutations. *JAMA Oncol* Published online June 30, 2016.

75. Moore KN, Fader AN. Uterine papillary serous carcinoma. *Clin*

Obstet Gynecol 2011; 54(2): 278-291.

76. Jemal A, Bray F, Center MM, Ferlay J, Ward E, Forman D. Global cancer statistics. *CA Cancer J Clin* 2011; 61: 69–90.

77. Jemal A, Siegel R, Xu J, Ward E. Cancer statistics, 2010. *CA Cancer J Clin* 2010: 10.3322/caac.20073.

78. Prostate Cancer UK, http://prostatecanceruk.org/prostate-information/about-prostate-cancer. Accessed Jun 2017.

79. IMPACT, http://impact-study.co.uk/public/aboutprostatecancer. Accessed Mar 2016.

80. Castro E, Goh C, Olmos D. Germline BRCA mutations are associated with higher risk of nodal involvement, distant metastasis, and poor survival outcomes in prostate cancer. *J Clin Oncol* 2013; 31: 1748–1757.

81. Edwards SM, Evans DG, Hope Q. Prostate cancer in BRCA2 germline mutation carriers is associated with poorer prognosis. *Br J Cancer* 2010; 103: 918–924.

82. Gallagher DJ, Gaudet MM, Pal P. Germline BRCA mutations denote a clinicopathologic subset of prostate cancer. *Clin Cancer Res* 2010; 16: 2115–2121.

83. Mitra A, Fisher C, Foster CS. Prostate cancer in male BRCA1 and BRCA2 mutation carriers has a more aggressive phenotype. *Br J Cancer* 2008; 98: 502–507.

84. Thorne H, Willems AJ, Niedermayr E. Decreased prostate cancer-specific survival of men with BRCA2 mutations from multiple breast cancer families. *Cancer Prev Res* 2011; 4: 1002–1010.

85. Tryggvadottir L, Vidarsdottir L, Thorgeirsson T. Prostate cancer progression and survival in BRCA2 mutation carriers. *J Natl Cancer Inst.* 2007; 99: 929–935.

86. www.nhs.uk/Conditions/Cancer-of-the-pancreas/Pages/Causes. aspx. Accessed Jun 2016.

87. Pancreatic Cancer UK, www.pancreaticcancer.org.uk/information-and-support/facts-about-pancreatic-cancer/risk-factors-for-pancreatic-cancer/. Accessed Dec 2016.

88. Cancer Research UK, www.cancerresearchuk.org/health-professional/cancer-statistics/statistics-by-cancer-type/pancreatic-cancer/survival. Accessed Dec 2016.

89. www.pancreatic.org/site/c.htJYJ8MPIwE/b.891917/k.5123/ Prognosis_of_Pancreatic_Cancer.htm. Accessed Dec 2016.

90. Cancer Research UK, www.cancerresearchuk.org/health-professional/cancer-statistics/statistics-by-cancer-type/pancreatic-cancer/incidence#ref1. Accessed Feb 2017.

91. Van Asperen CJ, Brohet R, Meijers-Heijboer E et al. Cancer risks in BRCA2 families: estimates for sites other than breast and ovary. *J Med Genet.* 2005;42(9): 711-719.

92. Friedenson B. BRCA1 and BRCA2 pathways and the risk of cancers other than breast or ovarian. *MedGenMed* 2005; 7(2): 60.

93. Risch HA, McLaughlin JR, Cole DE et al. Population BRCA1 and BRCA2 mutation frequencies and cancer penetrances: a kin-cohort study in Ontario, Canada. *J Natl Cancer Inst* 2006; 98(23): 1694-1706.

94. Canto MI, Harinck F, Hruban RH et al. International Cancer of the Pancreas Screening (CAPS) Consortium summit on the management of patients with increased risk for familial pancreatic cancer. *Gut* 2013; 62(3): 339-347.

95. http://emedicine.medscape.com/article/2246978-overview, Pancreatic Cancer Guidelines, Pancreatic cancer guidelines. Accessed Dec 2016.

96. www.nhs.uk/Conditions/Malignant-melanoma/Pages/Introduction.aspx. Skin cancer (melanoma). Accessed Sep 2016.

97. Skin Cancer Foundation, www.skincancer.org/skin-cancer-information/melanoma. Melanoma. Accessed Sep 2016.

98. Cancer Research UK, www.cancerresearchuk.org/about-cancer/causes-of-cancer/inherited-cancer-genes-and-increased-cancer-risk/inherited-genes-and-cancer-types#inherited_genes3. Accessed Dec 2016.

99. Gumaste PV, Penn LA, Cymerman RM et al. Skin cancer risk in BRCA1/2 mutation carriers. *Br J Dermatol* 2015; 172(6): 1498-1506.

100. Ginsburg OM, Kim-Sing C, Foulkes WD, Ghadirian P, Lynch HT, Sun P, Narod SA; Hereditary Breast Cancer Clinical Study Group. BRCA1 and BRCA2 families and the risk of skin cancer. *Fam Cancer* 2010; 9(4): 489-493.

101. Harbour JW. The genetics of uveal melanoma: an emerging framework for targeted therapy. *Pigment Cell Melanoma Res* 2012; 25(2): 171–181.

102. Liede A, Karlan BY, Narod SA. Cancer risks for male carriers of germline mutations in BRCA1 or BRCA2: a review of the literature. *J Clin Oncol* 2004; 22(4): 735-742.

103. www.dailymail.co.uk/femail/article-2709950/Generation-

tanners-spike-deadly-melanoma.html, 'Tanned skin is damaged skin': Surgeon general warns sun-loving Americans after 200% spike in deadly melanoma. Accessed Sep 2016.

104. www.skincancer.org/skin-cancer-information/skin-cancer-facts. Accessed Oct 2015.

105. Lubinski J, Phelan CM, Ghadirian P et al. Cancer variation associated with the position of the mutation in the BRCA2 gene. *Fam Cancer* 2004; 3(1): 1-10.

106. Breast Cancer Linkage Consortium. Cancer risks in BRCA2 mutation carriers. *J Natl Cancer Inst* 1999; 91(15): 1310-1316.

107. Wang Y et al. Rare variants of large effect in BRCA2 and CHEK2 affect risk of lung cancer. *Nature Genetics* 2014; 46: 736-741.

Section IV: Managing your risk

1. Warner E, Plewes DB, Hill KA et.al. Surveillance of BRCA1 and BRCA2 mutation carriers with magnetic resonance imaging, ultrasound, mammography, and clinical breast examination. *JAMA* 2004; 292(11): 1317-1325.

2. The Royal Marsden Hospital, www.royalmarsden.nhs.uk/sites/default/files/files_trust/brca_0.pdf – The Royal Marsden's: A Beginner's Guide to BRCA1 and BRCA2. Accessed Dec 2016.

3. Cancer Research UK, www.cancerresearchuk.org/about-cancer/find-a-clinical-trial/a-study-comparing-digital-breast-tomosynthesis-standard-mammogram-screening-younger-high-risk-women#undefined. Accessed Feb 2017.

4. Cancer Research UK, www.cancerresearchuk.org/sites/default/files/breast-screening-review-exec_0.pdf. Accessed Feb 2017.

5. www.radiologyinfo.org/en/info.cfm?pg=dense-breasts, Dense breasts. Accessed Feb 2017.

6. Breast Density-Breast cancer screening Brochure, ACR-SBI, www.acr.org/~/media/ACR/Documents/PDF/QualitySafety/Resources/Breast-Imaging/Breast-Density-bro_ACR_SBI_F.pdf. Accessed Jan 2017.

7. www.breastcancer.org/risk/factors/dense_breasts. Accessed Dec 2016.

8. http://drattai.com/areas-of-focus/dense-breast-tissue/. Accessed Dec 2016.

9.   McCormack VA, Dos Santos Silva I. Breast density and parenchymal patterns as markers of breast cancer risk: a meta-analysis. *Cancer Epidemiol Biomark Prev Publ Am Assoc Cancer Res Cosponsored Am Soc Prev Oncol* 2006; 15(6): 1159–1169.

10. Passaperuma K, Warner E, Hill KA et al. Is mammographic breast density a breast cancer risk factor in women with BRCA mutations? *J Clin Oncol* 2010; 28(23): 3779-3783.

11. Pruthi S, Gostout BS, Lindor NM. Identification and Management of Women with BRCA Mutations or Hereditary Predisposition for Breast and Ovarian Cancer. *Mayo Clin Proc* 2010; 85(12): 1111–1120.

12. http://breast-cancer.ca/densitbi-rads/, Breast Density classifications according to the BI-RADS lexicon, March 10, 2016 By Steven Halls. Accessed Mar 2016.

13. http://acsh.org/news/2016/09/07/both-doctors-and-patients-confused-dense-breasts-9960. Both Doctors and Patients confused By Dense Breasts. Accessed Sep 2016.

14. www.healthywomen.org/content/ask-expert/1285/breast-density. Accessed Jul 2015.

15. Evans DG, Gaarenstroom KN, Stirling D et al. Screening for familial ovarian cancer: Poor survival of BRCA1/2 related cancers. *Journal of Medical Genetics* 2009; 46(9): 593–597.

16. Cancer Research UK, www.cancerresearchuk.org/about-cancer/type/ovarian-cancer/diagnosis/ovarian-cancer-tests#blood. Accessed Feb 2017.

17. Jacobs IJ, Menon U, Ryan A et al. Ovarian cancer screening and mortality in the UK Collaborative Trial of Ovarian Cancer Screening (UKCTOCS): a randomised controlled trial. *Lancet* 2016; 387: 945-956.

18. Menon U, Gentry-Maharaj A, Burnell M et al. Ovarian cancer population screening and mortality after long-term follow-up in the UK Collaborative Trial of Ovarian Cancer Screening (UKCTOCS): a randomised controlled trial. *Lancet* 2021; 397(10290): 2182-2193. DOI:https://doi.org/10.1016/S0140-6736(21)00731-5

19. Cancer Research UK, www.cancerresearchuk.org/about-cancer/find-a-clinical-trial/a-study-looking-at-ovarian-cancer-screening-for-women-at-high-risk-the-united-kingdom-familial-ovarian-cancer-screening-study#undefined. Accessed Mar 2017.

20. The Eve Appeal, https://eveappeal.org.uk/our-research/our-

research-programmes/ukfocss/. Accessed Feb 2017.

21. Rosenthal AN, Fraser LS, Philpott S et al. Evidence of Stage Shift in Women Diagnosed With Ovarian Cancer During Phase II of the United Kingdom Familial Ovarian Cancer Screening Study. *J Clin Oncol* 2017; 27. doi: 10.1200/JCO.2016.69.9330.

22. Djulbegovic M, Beyth RJ, Neuberger MM, Stoffs TL, Vieweg J, Djulbegovic B, Dahm P. Screening for prostate cancer: systematic review and meta-analysis of randomized controlled trials. *BMJ* 2010; 341: c4543. doi:10.1136/bmj.c4543. PMC 2939952. PMID 20843937.

23. Bancroft EK, Page EC, Castro E, et al. Targeted prostate cancer screening in BRCA1 and BRCA2 mutation carriers: results from the initial screening round of the IMPACT study. *Eur Urol* 2014; 66: 489–499.

24. King MC, Wieand S, Hale K, et al. Tamoxifen and breast cancer incidence among women with inherited mutations in BRCA1 and BRCA2: National Surgical Adjuvant Breast and Bowel Project (nsabp-p1) Breast Cancer Prevention Trial. *JAMA* 2001; 286 (18):2251-2256.

25. Phillips KA, Milne RL, Rookus MA, et al. Tamoxifen and risk of contralateral breast cancer for BRCA1 and BRCA2 mutation carriers. *Journal of Clinical Oncology* 2013; 31(25): 3091-3099.

26. Beiner ME, Finch A, Rosen B, et al. The risk of endometrial cancer in women with BRCA1 and BRCA2 mutations. A prospective study. *Gynecol Oncol.* 2007 Jan;104(1):7-10.

27. Guidance for the Management of Breast Cancer Treatment-Induced Bone Loss, A consensus position statement from a UK Expert Group. National Osteoporosis Society. https://nos.org.uk/media/98027/bone-health-guidelines-breast-cancer-treatments.pdf. Accessed Nov 2015.

28. McLaughlin JR, Risch HA, Lubinski J et al. Reproductive risk factors for ovarian cancer in carriers of BRCA1 or BRCA2 mutations: A case-control study. *Lancet Oncology* 2007; 8 (1): 26-34.

29. Whittemore AS, Balise RR, Pharoah PD et al. Oral contraceptive use and ovarian cancer risk among carriers of BRCA1 or BRCA2 mutations. *Br J Cancer* 2004; 91: 1911–1915.

30. Narod SA, Risch H, Moslehi R et al. Oral contraceptives and the risk of hereditary ovarian cancer. Hereditary Ovarian Cancer

Clinical Study Group. *N Engl J Med* 1998; 339: 424–428.

31. Moorman PG, Havrilesky LJ, Gierisch JM et al. Oral contraceptives and risk of ovarian cancer and breast cancer among high-risk women: a systematic review and meta-analysis. *J Clin Oncol* 2013; 31: 4188–4198.

32. Domchek SM, Friebel TM et al. Association of risk-reducing surgery in BRCA1 or BRCA2 mutation carriers with cancer risk and mortality. *JAMA* 2010; 304 (9): 967-975.

33. www.telegraph.co.uk/women/health/surgical-menopause-linked-to-poor-memory-and-early-onset-dementi/, 'Surgical menopause' linked to poor memory and early-onset dementia. By India Sturgis, 27 July 2016. Accessed Jul 2016.

34. Rebbeck TR, Lynch HT, Neuhausen SL et al. Prophylactic Oophorectomy in Carriers of BRCA1 or BRCA2 Mutations. *N Engl J Med* 2002; 346:1616-1622.

35. Rebbeck TR, Kauff ND, Domchek SM. Meta-analysis of risk reduction estimates associated with risk-reducing salpingo-oophorectomy in BRCA1 or BRCA2 mutation carriers. *J Natl Cancer Inst* 2009; 101(2):80-87.

36. Domchek SM, Weber BL. Clinical management of BRCA1 and BRCA2 mutation carriers. *Oncogene* 2006; 25, 5825–5831.

37. Sidon L, Ingham A, Clancy T et al. Uptake of risk-reducing salpingo-oophorectomy in women carrying a BRCA1 or BRCA2 mutation: evidence for lower uptake in women affected by breast cancer and older women. *British Journal of Cancer* 2012; 106: 775–779.

38. Finch AP, Lubinski J, Møller P et al. Impact of oophorectomy on cancer incidence and mortality in women with a BRCA1 or BRCA2 mutation. *J Clin Oncol* 2014; 32: 1547–1553.

39. Greene MH, Mai PL, Schwartz PE. Does bilateral salpingectomy with ovarian retention warrant consideration as a temporary bridge to risk-reducing bilateral oophorectomy in BRCA1/2 mutation carriers? *Am J Obstet Gynecol* 2011; 204: 19.e1–6.

40. Society of Gynecologic Oncology. SGO Clinical Practice Statement: Salpingectomy for ovarian cancer prevention. www.sgo.org/clinical-practice/guidelines/sgo-clinical-practice-statement-salpingectomy-for-ovarian-cancer-prevention/. Accessed Jul 2016.

41. Gilks CB, Miller D. Opportunistic salpingectomy for women at low risk for development of ovarian cancer: the time has come. *Gynecol*

Oncol 2013; 129: 443–444.

42. Kwon JS, Tinker A, Pansegrau G, McAlpine J, Housty M, McCullum M, Gilks CB. Prophylactic salpingectomy and delayed oophorectomy as an alternative for BRCA mutation carriers. *Obstet Gynecol* 2013; 121(1): 14-24.

43. www.nhs.uk/Conditions/Menopause/Pages/Symptoms.aspx. Accessed Dec 2016.

44. Colditz GA, Willett WC, Stampfer MJ et al. Menopause and the risk of coronary heart disease in women. *N Engl J Med* 1987; 316: 1105–1110.

45. Melton LJ, 3rd, Khosla S, Malkasian GD et al. Fracture risk after bilateral oophorectomy in elderly women. *J Bone Miner Res* 2003; 18(5): 900–905.

46. Marchetti C, Iadarola R, Palaia I, di Donato V, Perniola G, Muzii L, Panici PB. Hormone therapy in oophorectomized BRCA1/2 mutation carriers. *Menopause.* 2014; 21(7): 763-768.

47. The Hysterectomy Association, www.hysterectomy-association. org.uk/information/the-menopause/osteoporosis-and-the-menopause/ Osteoporosis and the menopause. Accessed Apr 2016.

48. Tucker PE, et al. Prevalence of sexual dysfunction after risk-reducing salpingo-oophorectomy. *Gynecol Oncol* 2016; 140(1): 95-100.

49. NICE Guideline NG23, www.nice.org.uk/guidance/ng23, Menopause: diagnosis and management. Published date Nov 2015.

50. Fang CY, Cherry C, Devarajan K, Li T, Malick J, Daly MB. A prospective study of quality of life among women undergoing risk-reducing salpingo-oophorectomy versus gynecologic screening for ovarian cancer. *Gynecol Oncol* 2009; 112(3): 594-600.

51. Kotsopoulos J, Lubinski J, Neuhausen SL et al. Weight gain after oophorectomy among women with a BRCA1 or BRCA2 mutation. *Womens' Health* (Lond Engl) 2015; 11(4): 453-459.

52. Hallowell N, Mackay J, Richards M, Gore M, Jacobs I. High-risk premenopausal women's experiences of undergoing prophylactic oophorectomy: a descriptive study. *Genet Test* 2004; 8: 148–156.

53. Kauff ND, Hurley KE, Hensley ML et al. Ovarian carcinoma screening in women at intermediate risk: impact on quality of life and need for invasive follow-up. *Cancer* 2005; 104: 314–320.

54. Michelsen TM, Dørum A, Tropé CG, Osså SD, Dahl AA. Fatigue

and quality of life after risk-reducing salpingo-oophorectomy in women at increased risk for hereditarybreast-ovarian cancer. *Int J Gynecol Cancer* 2009; 19(6): 1029-1036.

55. The Telegraph, www.telegraph.co.uk/women/health/surgical-menopause-linked-to-poor-memory-and-early-onset-dementi/. Accessed Sep 2016.

56. Suberbielle E, Djukic B, Evans M et al. DNA repair factor BRCA1 depletion occurs in Alzheimer brains and impairs cognitive function in mice. *Nature Communications* 2015; 6: 8897. doi:10.1038/ncommms9897

57. Matthews KA, Meilahn E, Kuller LH, Kelsey SF, Caggiula AW, Wing RR. Menopause and risk factors for coronary heart disease. *N Engl J Med* 1989; 321(10): 641–646.

58. www.cardiosmart.org/News-and-Events/2013/05/Removal-of-Uterus-and-Ovaries-Does-Not-Increase-Heart-Disease-Risk-in-Women. Accessed Oct 2015.

59. www.heart.org/HEARTORG/Conditions/More/MyHeartandStrokeNews/Menopause-and-Heart-Disease_UCM_448432_Article.jsp#.WCXBgfXXKHs, Menopause and Heart Disease. Accessed Nov 2016.

60. Manning AT et al. Nipple-sparing mastectomy in patients with BRCA1/2 mutations and variants of uncertain significance. *Br J Surg* 2015; 102(11): 1354-1359.

61. Metcalfe KA et al. Long-Term Psychosocial Functioning in Women with Bilateral Prophylactic Mastectomy: Does Preservation of the Nipple-Areolar Complex Make a Difference? *Ann Surg Oncol* 2015; 22(10): 3324-3330.

62. Dossett LA et al. Prospective evaluation of skin and nipple-areola sensation and patient satisfaction after nipple-sparing mastectomy. *J Surg Oncol* 2016; 114(1): 11-16.

63. Frost MH, Schaid DJ, Sellers TA et al. Long-term satisfaction and psychological and social function following bilateral prophylactic mastectomy. *JAMA* 2000; 284(3): 319-324.

64. Brandberg Y, Sandelin K, Erikson S et al. Psychological reactions, quality of life, and body image after bilateral prophylactic mastectomy in women at high risk for breast cancer: a prospective 1-year follow-up study. *J Clin Oncol* 2008; 26(24): 3943-3949.

65. www.sharecare.com/health/breast-cancer/what-is-post-

mastectomy-pain-syndrome. What is post-mastectomy pain syndrome? Accessed Oct 2016.

66. Gahm J, Wickman M, Brandberg Y. Bilateral prophylactic mastectomy in women with inherited risk of breast cancer-- prevalence of pain and discomfort, impact on sexuality, quality of life and feelings of regret two years after surgery. *Breast* 2010; 19(6): 462-469.

67. Rodriguez-Feliz J, et al. Embrace the Change: Incorporating Single-Stage Implant Breast Reconstruction into Your Practice. *Plast Reconstr Surg* 2015; 136(2): 221-231.

68. www.the-cosmetic-surgery-directory.com/article_implantmuscle. html, Breast Implants Over the Muscle vs. Under the Muscle, By Jennifer Kimberley. Accessed Sep 2016.

69. Breast Implants. Information for women considering breast implants, April 2011, Medicines and Healthcare products Regulatory Agency (MHRA). Accessed Sep 2016.

70. The European Commission and its Scientific Committee on Health, Environmental and Emerging Risks. FINAL Opinion on the safety of breast implants in relation to anaplastic large cell lymphoma. The European Commission. 26 March 2021. https://ec.europa.eu/ health/sites/default/files/scientific_committees/scheer/docs/ scheer_o_018.pdf. Accessed June 2021.

71. Kurian AW, Sigal BM, Plevritis SK. Survival analysis of cancer risk reduction strategies for BRCA1/2 mutation carriers. *J Clin Oncol* 2010; 28(2): 222-231.

72. Cancer Research UK, http://scienceblog.cancerresearchuk. org/2010/04/07/fruit-vegetables-and-cancer-why-its-still-worth-getting-your-five-a-day/. Accessed Mar 2017.

73. Nkondjock A, Robidoux A, Paredes Y, Narod SA, Ghadirian P. Diet, lifestyle and BRCA-related breast cancer risk among French-Canadians. *Breast Cancer Res Treat* 2006; 98(3): 285-294.

74. Pruthi S, Gostout BS, Lindor NM. Identification and Management of Women with BRCA Mutations or Hereditary Predisposition for Breast and Ovarian Cancer. *Mayo Clin Proc* 2010; 85(12): 1111–1120.

75. Cancer Research UK, www.cancerresearchuk.org/about-cancer/ type/ovarian-cancer/about/ovarian-cancer-risks-and-causes. Accessed Sep 2015.

76. McTiernan A, Kooperberg C, White E et al. Recreational physical

activity and the risk of breast cancer in postmenopausal women: the Women's Health Initiative Cohort Study. *JAMA* 2003; 290(10): 1331-1336.

77. Reeves GK, Pirie K, Beral V, Green J, Spencer E, Bull D. Cancer incidence and mortality in relation to body mass index in the Million Women Study: cohort study. *BMJ* 2007; 335(7630): 1134.

78. Carpenter CL, Ross RK, Paganini-Hill A et al. Effect of family history, obesity and exercise on breast cancer risk among postmenopausal women. *Int J Cancer* 2003; 106(1): 96-102.

79. King MC, Marks JH, Mandell JB. New York Breast Cancer Study Group. Breast and ovarian cancer risks due to inherited mutations in BRCA1 and BRCA2. *Science* 2003; 302(5645): 643-646.

80. Friedenreich CM, Neilson HK, O'Reilly R et al. Effects of a High vs Moderate Volume of Aerobic Exercise on Adiposity Outcomes in Postmenopausal Women: A Randomized Clinical Trial. *JAMA Oncol* 2015; 1(6): 766-776.

80a. Park A. Here's the amount of exercise that lowers breast cancer risk. *Time* 16 July 2015. http://time.com/3960035/exercise-breast-cancer (Accessed 10 Sep 2017.)

81. www.cancer.org/cancer/breastcancer/detailedguide/breast-cancer-risk-factors. Accessed Dec 2016.

82. Secretan B, Straif K, Baan R, et al. A review of human carcinogens-Part E: tobacco, areca nut, alcohol, coal smoke, and salted fish. *Lancet Oncol* 2009; 10: 1033-1034.

83. Parkin DM et al. Cancers attributable to the consumption of alcohol in the UK in 2010. *Br J Cancer* 2011; 106(S2): S14-S18.

84. Dorgan JF, Baer DJ, Albert PS, et al. Serum hormones and the alcohol-breast cancer association in postmenopausal women. *J Natl Cancer Inst* 2001; 93: 710-715.

85. Dennis J, Krewski D, Cote FS et al. Breast cancer risk in relation to alcohol consumption and BRCA gene mutations--a case-only study of gene-environment interaction. *Breast J* 2011; 17(5): 477–484.

86. McDonald JA, Goyal A, Terry MB. Alcohol Intake and Breast Cancer Risk: Weighing the Overall Evidence. *Curr Breast Cancer Rep.* 2013; 5(3): doi:10.1007/s12609-013-0114-z.

87. McGuire V, John EM, Felberg A et al. No increased risk of breast cancer associated with alcohol consumption among carriers of BRCA1 and BRCA2 mutations ages <50 years. Cancer

epidemiology, biomarkers & prevention : a publication of the *American Association for Cancer Research*, cosponsored by the *American Society of Preventive Oncology* 2006; 15(8): 1565–1567.

88. Dennis J, Ghadirian P, Little J et al. Alcohol consumption and the risk of breast cancer among BRCA1 and BRCA2 mutation carriers. *Breast* 2010; 19(6): 479–483.

89. Lecarpentier J, Nogues C, Mouret-Fourme E et al. Variation in breast cancer risk with mutation position, smoking, alcohol, and chest X-ray history, in the French National BRCA1/2 carrier cohort (GENEPSO) *Breast Cancer Research and Treatment* 2011; 130(3): 927–938.

90. Cybulski C, Lubinski J, Huzarski T. Prospective evaluation of alcohol consumption and the risk of breast cancer in BRCA1 and BRCA2 mutation carriers. *Breast Cancer Research and Treatment* 2015; 151(2): 435-441.

91. www.nice.org.uk/guidance/cg164. Accessed Dec 2016.

92. Cancer Research UK, www.cancerresearchuk.org/about-cancer/ causes-of-cancer/smoking-and-cancer/how-smoking-causes-cancer. Accessed Apr 2016.

93. Breastcancer.org, www.breastcancer.org/risk/factors/smoking. Accessed Apr 2016.

94. Nkondjock A, Robidoux A, Paredes Y, Narod SA, Ghadirian P. Diet, lifestyle and BRCA-related breast cancer risk among French-Canadians. *Breast Cancer Res Treat* 2006; 98(3): 285-294.

95. Ghadirian P, Lubinski J, Lynch H et al. Smoking and the risk of breast cancer among carriers of BRCA mutations. *Int J Cancer* 2004; 110: 413–416.

96. Ginsburg O, Ghadirian P, Lubinski J et al. Smoking and the risk of breast cancer in BRCA1 and BRCA2 carriers: an update. *Breast Cancer Research and Treatment* 2009; 114(1): 127–135.

97. Breast Cancer Family Registry, Kathleen Cuningham Consortium for Research into Familial Breast Cancer (Australasia), Ontario Cancer Genetics Network (Canada). Smoking and risk of breast cancer in carriers of mutations in BRCA1 or BRCA2 aged less than 50 years. *Breast Cancer Res Treat* 2008; 109(1): 67-75.

98. Passarelli MN, et al. Cigarette Smoking Before and After Breast Cancer Diagnosis: Mortality From Breast Cancer and Smoking-Related Diseases. *J Clin Oncol* 2016; 34: 1315–1322.

99. Faber MT, Kjær SK, Dehlendorff C et al. Cigarette smoking and risk of ovarian cancer: a pooled analysis of 21 case-control studies. *Cancer Causes Control* 2013; 24(5): 989-1004.

100. Wang Y et al. Rare variants of large effect in BRCA2 and CHEK2 affect risk of lung cancer. *Nature Genetics* 2014; 46, 736-741.

101. Michailidou K et al. Large-scale genotyping identifies 41 new loci associated with breast cancer risk. *Nat Genet* 2013; 45: 353-361.

102. Association of British Insurers (ABI). The Concordat and Moratorium on genetics and insurance 2014. www.abi.org.uk. Accessed Aug 2016.

103. National Health Service UK (NHS). www.organdonation.nhs.uk. Accessed Nov 2016.

104. www.theguardian.com/science/2015/may/10/crispr-genome-editing-dna-upgrade-technology-genetic-disease, Crispr: is it a good idea to 'upgrade' our DNA? By Zoe Corbyn, Sunday 10 May 2015, Accessed Sep 2016.

105. www.theguardian.com/science/2015/apr/23/scientists-genetically-modify-human-embryos-in-controversial-world-first, Ian Sample, science editor, Thursday 23 April 2015, Accessed Sep 2016.

106. www.bbc.co.uk/news/health-34202250, BBC News, CRISPR genome editing 'an important tool' 10 Sep 2015, Accessed Sep 2016.

Section V: My personal journey

1. Verstraelen H, Verhelst R, Vaneechoutte et al. Group A streptococcal vaginitis: an unrecognised cause of vaginal symptoms in adult women. *Arch Gynecol Obstet* 2011; 284(1): 95-98.

Resources

Websites for further information

This list of resources is intended to help you find further information or additional sources of support, but not all information will be relevant to all individuals:

National Institute for Health and Clinical Excellence (NICE), www.nice.org.uk – provides national guidance and advice to improve health and social care guidelines, including the CG164 on Familial breast cancer available at https://www.nice.org.uk/guidance/cg164.

Breastcancer.org, www.breastcancer.org/ – is a non-profit organisation dedicated to providing the most reliable, complete and up-to-date information about breast cancer.

The EMBRACE study, http://ccge.medschl.cam.ac.uk/embrace/ – a major study ongoing in the UK to examine lifestyle and additional genetic factors which may increase or decrease cancer risk in people who are known to carry a BRCA1 or BRCA2 gene mutation.

The Breast and Ovarian Cancer Susceptibility (BOCS) study, www.icr.ac.uk/our-research/research-divisions/division-of-genetics-and-epidemiology/genetic-susceptibility/research-projects/the-breast-and-ovarian-cancer-susceptibility-(bocs)-study – the purpose of this study is to identify the genetic factors involved in causing breast and ovarian cancer.

The IMPACT study, www.impact-study.co.uk/ – is an international study which aims to discover whether screening to detect prostate cancer can be targeted at men who carry the BRCA1, BRCA2 and Lynch Syndrome alterations, leading to earlier diagnosis and improved survival.

The UKCTOCS study website, www.ucl.ac.uk/womens-health/research/womens-cancer/gynaecological-cancer-research-centre/ukctocs – is the world's largest ovarian cancer screening trial looking at whether screening tests would be useful for diagnosing ovarian cancer in the general population and if screening can save lives.

The UK FOCSS website, www.ucl.ac.uk/womens-health/research/womens-cancer/gynaecological-cancer-research-centre/ukfocss – a UK study looking at ovarian cancer screening in high-risk women. The aim of this study was to find out which screening tests are best for women at high risk of ovarian cancer and to determine how often women should be screened.

Association of British Insurers (ABI), www.abi.org.uk – provides consumers with general information on insurance and savings products and services. The Concordat and Moratorium on Genetics and Insurance 2014 may be found on this website. Tel: 020 7600 3333.

Charities, support groups and other useful contacts

Cancer Research UK (CRUK), www.cruk.org.uk. Cancer Research UK is the world's largest cancer research organisation, outside the USA. If you have a question about cancer, and you are in the UK or Ireland, you can call their free phone helpline: 0808 800 40 40.

Macmillan Cancer Support, www.macmillan.org.uk. Macmillan's ambition is to reach and improve the lives of everyone living with cancer and to inspire millions of others to do the same. Free phone helpline: 0808 808 00 00.

The Eve Appeal – www.eveappeal.org.uk – For better detection and improved treatment of all five gynaecological cancers. They have a dedicated specialist gynaecological cancer information service called AskEve available on 0808 802 0019. Or, get in touch via email: nurse@eveappeal.org.uk

FORCE – Facing Our Risk of Cancer Empowered, www.facingourrisk.org – provides information and support to individuals and families affected by hereditary breast, ovarian and other cancers. FORCE's mission is to improve the lives of individuals and families affected by hereditary breast, ovarian and related cancers.

National Cancer Institute, www.cancer.gov – a detailed American site with information for both people with cancer and health professionals.

Facebook: there are several BRCA peer support groups on this social networking site www.facebook.com including, among others:

- Understanding BRCA – information and support group for BRCA mutation carriers and others in the HBOC community;

- BRCA Mutations Ireland and the UK – information and support for anyone affected by the BRCA1 and BRCA2 gene or other high-risk genetic mutations.

- BRCA Sisterhood – offers support for women with a BRCA gene mutation;

- BRCA Strong – sharing information with women on the BRCA gene and the risk-reducing options available;

- Mutant Strong! – offers support to BRCA mutation carriers and others in the HBOC community (women only);

- BRCA1 or BRCA2 Genetic Ovarian & Breast Cancer Gene – support group for individuals or their family members who are BRCA positive;

- BRCA Support – Surveillance – a support group for BRCA mutation carriers who are choosing surveillance over surgery;

- BRCA1/2 – supporting your loved ones – a support group for any family members who are supporting their loved ones with BRCA gene mutations;

- BRCA Advanced 101 & 102 Journal Club on Facebook – a group to foster knowledge and discussion via scientific studies and articles pertaining to high-risk population and/or BRCA community.

BrCa Umbrella Support and Social Network: an online support forum for BRCA carriers http://brcaumbrella.ning.com/

My Destiny Foundation, Inc. – is one of the leading Foundations for women at high risk for breast cancer due to family history or carriers of the BRCA gene mutation, www.mydestiny-us.com/index.html

Bright Pink – based in the US and is the only national non-profit organisation focused on prevention and early detection of breast and ovarian cancer in young women www.brightpink.org/

Pink Hope: an Australian website for BRCA carriers, www.pinkhope.org.au/ – is a preventative health organisation working to ensure every individual can assess, manage and reduce their risk of breast and ovarian cancer, providing every family the support they need.

Breast Cancer Now, http://breastcancernow.org/ – is the UK's largest breast cancer charity, created by the merger of Breast Cancer Campaign and Breakthrough Breast Cancer, funding research to help prevent, detect, treat and stop breast cancer.

Triple Negative Breast Cancer Foundation, www.tnbcfoundation.org/helpline/ – offers free, professional support services to patients, families and health providers coping with a diagnosis of triple negative breast cancer.

Young Survival Coalition (YSC), www.youngsurvival.org – an organisation for young women with breast cancer.

CancerCare, www.cancercare.org – free support service offering counselling, support groups, education and financial assistance.

Genetic Alliance UK, www.geneticalliance.org.uk – a national charity working to improve the lives of patients and families affected by all types of genetic conditions.

Hope for two the pregnant with cancer network, www.pregnantwithcancer.org/ – an organisation for women diagnosed with cancer while pregnant.

Flat & Fabulous, www.flatandfabulous.org/ – an organization committed to advocating and providing support for those who are living post mastectomy without reconstruction.

Living Beyond Breast Cancer (LBBC), www.lbbc.org – provides emotional and practical support for women diagnosed with breast cancer.

Shine Cancer Support, www.shinecancersupport.org/ – supports young adults in their 20s, 30s and 40s living with any type of cancer diagnosis.

The Willow Foundation, www.willowfoundation.org.uk/ – is a national charity that provides psychological and emotional support for seriously ill 16 to 40 year olds through the provision of special day experiences.

Breast Reconstruction Awareness (BRA) Group, Department of Plastic & Reconstructive Surgery, John Radcliffe Hospital, Oxford, England – their aim is to raise awareness about breast reconstruction and to provide support for all those involved. Email: oxfordbreastreconstruction@gmail.com

Men Against Breast Cancer – Caring about the women we love, www.menagainstbreastcancer.org – a non-profit organization designed to provide targeted support services that educate and empower men to be effective caregivers when cancer strikes. Email: info@menagainstbreastcancer.org

Target Ovarian Cancer, www.targetovariancancer.org.uk – is the UK's leading ovarian cancer charity which works to improve early diagnosis, fund life-saving research and provide much-needed support to women with ovarian cancer.

Ovacome ovarian cancer charity, www.ovacome.org.uk/ – a charity which operates an ovarian cancer helpline service by telephone (0800 008 7054) and email (ovacome@ovacome.org.uk), offering information and emotional support to women, their families, friends, and carers.

Ovarian Cancer Action, www.ovarian.org.uk – the UK's ovarian cancer research charity. Email: info@ovarian.org.uk

The Daisy Network, www.daisynetwork.org.uk/ – provides information and support to women diagnosed with Premature Ovarian Insufficiency, also known as Premature Menopause.

The Menopause Exchange, www.menopause-exchange.co.uk/ – provides information on menopausal symptoms and coping with the menopause using HRT, prescribed medicine alternatives to HRT, complementary therapies and medicines and health promotion advice including nutrition, exercise and self-help lifestyle measures.

The Hysterectomy Association, www.hysterectomy-association.org. uk – aims to provide clear, concise information about hysterectomy, women's health, the menopause and HRT for women undergoing, or planning to undergo, surgery.

The Male Breast Cancer Coalition, http://malebreastcancercoalition. org/ – a not-for-profit patient advocacy organization, bringing everyone together to educate the world about male breast cancer.

HIS Breast Cancer Awareness, www.hisbreastcancer.org/ – created to assist men and women (girlfriends, wives, sisters & brothers, mothers & fathers, and friends), health care professionals, and anyone who is interested in learning about the risk, treatment(s), emotional aspect and stigmatism of men dealing with this disease.

Prostate Cancer UK, www.prostatecanceruk.org – offers information and support to anyone with concerns about prostate cancer. Offers a helpline and leaflets and funds research into prostate cancer. Email: info@prostatecanceruk.org

Helpline: 0800 074 8383.

Prostate Cancer Support Federation, www.tackleprostate.org – offers a helpline, website and campaigns under the name Tackle Prostate Cancer. Helpline: 0800 035 5302.

The National Osteoporosis Society (NOS), www.nos.org.uk/ – the only UK wide charity dedicated to ending the pain and suffering caused by osteoporosis. Helpline: 0808 800 0035.

Skin Cancer Foundation, www.skincancer.org/ - is the only international organization devoted solely to education, prevention, early detection, and prompt treatment of the world's most common cancer.

Melanoma UK, www.melanomauk.org.uk/ – a patient organisation dedicated to helping skin cancer patients during all stages and fundraising to provide melanoma nurses and research.

British Skin Foundation, Leading the fight against skin disease and skin cancer, http://britishskinfoundation.org.uk – the UK's only charity dedicated to skin research.

Index

Index

Index

Index

Index

Index

Also from Hammersmith Health Books

RECOVERY FROM INJURY, SURGERY AND INFECTION
A Nature Cures Book

By Nat H Hawes

Author of *Nature Cures: the A to Z of Ailments and Natural Foods*
and www.naturecures.co.uk

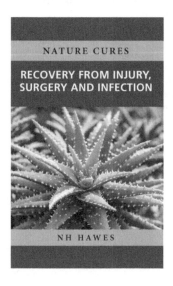

A practical guide to the foods richest in the nutrients required
for healing and fighting infection, including an A to Z of over
200 naturally antimicrobial plants, their active ingredients, the
conditions they have traditionally been used for and what the
latest research findings tell us about their properties.